TRAUMA INTEGRATED

HOW PRIMITIVE REFLEXES AND YOGA CAN SETTLE THE SCORE

VERONIKA PEÑA DE LA JARA

DISCLAIMER

The information presented in this book is for educational and informational purposes only. It is not intended to be a substitute for proper diagnosis and treatment by a licensed professional. If you have any questions about whether the information and advice presented in this book is suitable for you, please check with your trusted physician or healthcare provider. It is your responsibility to discern what of the information provided is useful for your health and to use it in appropriate and common-sense ways. The information is to be used at your own risk. The publisher and author disclaim any liabilities for any loss of profit, commercial or personal damages resulting from the use of information in this book.

DEDICATION

This book is dedicated to my beautiful, clever and intuitive friend Nicole Zimbler, without whom none of this work would have come about. My heart is full of gratitude for everything we have learnt and experienced together these past 25 years.

I dedicate this book also to my mother and father, without whom I would not exist. Thank you for taking a leap in love and creating me. The debt of gratitude can never be paid to those who give us life!

I have many supporters, cheer leaders and friends who have sustained me over many years, through many hardships and suffering. I am forever grateful for their support.

Finally, I am especially grateful to S N Goenka of the Vipassana Institute. Without his bringing his lineage of learning from Burma to India and to the West, my level of insight, wisdom and ethics would not be what they are. Always with so much Metta to you.

CONTENTS

INTRODUCTION

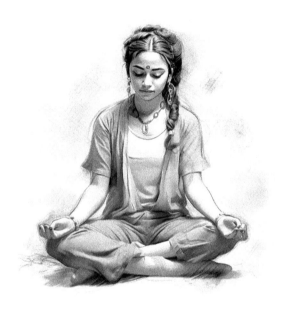

This book is about bringing life-transforming knowledge to the world, to humankind. In the course of my work thus far, I have come across a method that will help anyone out of Fight or Flight, Stress and Trauma. This book is for you, if you have always wondered how everyone around you manages to thrive in the face of fear of transforming themselves, or stepping up for what they believe in. It is also a book for yoga practitioners who wonder why their body always seems to go back to the old stress mode patterns only hours after their practice.

How would you feel if you knew there was a way to regularly and easily bring yourself back to your best self? If you learn about the nervous system and how you can manage it and change its modes of operation, you will be able to self-regulate and break free of all that is holding you back. Here, you will learn simple, short movements in the body that reset the nervous system and automatically bring it back to Rest and Digest function, out of trauma.

This work has been a very long journey. It began with the very first curious questions into what the Reflexes are when my son was a baby; to today, 13 years of work later. The work has been both by me on the mat, through observation in yoga practice of others, as well as intellectual learning of neurological functions as we understand them today. From baby yoga to adults' classes, from children to working with the SEN community, week after week, day after day, class after class for 25 years, this methodology and practice has been refined and reworked on the mat.

Nicole and I first met at my very first yoga class on Sairee Beach in Koh Tao, Thailand, in 1997. At this time, Koh Tao was a backwater on the backpacking trail in Thailand, mainly for those who wanted to learn to dive. It was hardly developed, being mostly a coconut plantation. Most accommodation was wooden huts, and the electrics went off at midnight. We were closely attuned to the moonlight as a result and I was working in a dive shop as a divemaster, diving 3 to 5 times a day. It was a paradise, now sadly lost to tourism. But there was something about diving, no doubt the ability to hear your breath when underwater, that led to a raising of my mid-twenties awareness and subsequently to attending my first yoga class.

I had never done anything like yoga before and I turned up to the class because as a Divemaster (more a guide really), I had developed a very tight body at the age of 27. I had recently attended a 7-day morning Chi Gong class and alongside diving itself, it had opened my eyes to a more mindful life; and I was curious to try more. I really had no idea what yoga was, but I went anyway, as I was told it was a good thing to do, not too dissimilar to Chi Gong. Our teacher had arrived on the island, printed up a load of posters and stuck them to the palm trees. Only Nicole and I turned up. She had decided to do 10 continuous days of yoga class every day for 2 hours. A bit of a baptism of fire for my poor old hamstrings! I will never forget the first time I managed to do a Yoga Nidra; I think I woke up as another person!

After 10 days I was hooked. I felt I had found my calling and have practised yoga ever since – for many months with Nicole in my room on Koh Tao. Then on returning to England 6 months later, we both decided to become teachers but in much different disciplines.

I first came across the Reflexes through a conversation I had with Nicole at Santosa Yoga Camp in 2011. Although Nicole and I had known each other for nearly 15 years at this point and we'd both become teachers at the same time, I was vaguely aware of what she was up to yoga-wise, as I had moved to rural Herefordshire and was committed to my teaching locally. I had had two more children and my youngest was now 9 months old and was starting to bum shuffle, a little late, but he was moving. Nicole casually mentioned that bum shuffling was something we wanted to avoid in babies and that she knew a few things that could help. She showed me 4 or 5 reflex moves which I did for the next few days. I was very much surprised when my son began to crawl a few days later. It was nothing short of a miracle, as far as I was concerned. Nicole had explained to me why missing out on crawling was not to be encouraged and like any mother, I was keen to see him crawl now I knew. I was immensely surprised, however, when it happened so quickly. To say my curiosity was piqued is an understatement! Now I wanted to know everything. I was teaching 4 baby yoga classes a week at various children's centres across Herefordshire at this point in my yoga career, and I felt that I needed to incorporate what I was learning into my classes, as I could see that it would benefit many of the babies I worked with. Many of the cohorts I was teaching were children of very deprived neighbourhoods with little resources and a lot of birth trauma. There were high percentages of caesarean sections and little awareness of child development. Over the next few years, there was a lot of reading and training that ensued; but really, Nicole was the fountain of my knowledge, as I systematically picked her brains coming back with case studies and real-time situations that I needed help with. It wasn't long before all my baby yoga classes included Reflex Integration work and they were very popular.

I remember one case; a lovely lady who came with her infant during her maternity leave. She worked at the local A Level college and was only one of two members of the faculty. She was very soon called back to work as the department was falling apart without her. What was interesting about her case was that a few months later, she took Friday mornings off work and re-joined Baby Yoga because her son was commando crawling; and she now knew he needed to be on all fours and cross crawling. He was over one year old and hadn't progressed since he'd started to get around by dragging himself across the floor. He was very fast but was obviously not using the left side of his body – later, we will explain what this meant; but after only a couple of weeks, he was up on his hands and knees and crawling everywhere. She returned to work, and I never saw them again. This story shows just how much of an impact Reflex Integration work can have on a baby, especially if at the time they should be integrating a particular reflex. The work then happens very fast and is particularly satisfying to work with.

It wasn't long before my curious mind started to wonder what effect this could have on general yoga classes. I was beginning to experience changes in my own body which were making me think that of course, it's only logical that it could affect how your body moves during practice.

My Monday night yoga class was my first class after a weekend of bodywork; and every week, as I began the Sun Salutations, I would find my hamstrings tight, and my back twinged from 2 days off stretching. By this point, I had been a yoga teacher for 12 years and still nothing much had changed when beginning class on Mondays. I always started Monday yoga class with some stiffness, and I thought it was normal to do so. However, after a few months of personal Reflex Yoga work, I began to find that I no longer stepped onto the mat and had so much work to do in this area. The whole of my lower body was mostly relaxed and if not, very quickly became so. It was as if it had remembered something from long ago where I could walk upon the earth without tension following from behind. Like a blueprint that I had returned to, where my body remembered how to be, naturally.

I had one student in class who had been coming to Monday night yoga class with me for 10 years. D was very enthusiastic and was a regular attendee, but she suffered greatly with her hamstrings and back. Every week, she arrived and her back and hamstrings were as bad as they had been every other Monday for over 10 years. There was an improvement over the duration of the class but once Monday swung around, we were back where we always started.

It was on one of these Mondays that I decided to go for it, and bring in some Reflex Integration moves which I had been practising with my babies in Baby Yoga. After one or two of these moves, the rest of the class continued with our usual stretching, but D stayed lying on the floor. After a while, I went over to make sure she was OK and she beamed at me from the floor and said, "I've never been so relaxed in my life. Can I just stay here and enjoy it for a while longer?" Of course, I walked away astounded. How could it be that after 10 years, this was the first time she had truly relaxed?

I couldn't quite believe the power of this method, and at that moment, I decided I was going to develop it into a full-blown method for adults. D's hamstrings and back problems began to improve and over the next 6 months there was more movement than there had been in the previous 10 years. I felt I was onto something...

I started to get excited that a Reflex Yoga method was possible and that I could investigate developing it. And as I had more time and more adult classes, I took on this mission with a fury. Not long after this development, Nicole and I founded Yotism, but our initial focus was on creating the Yoga for Autism Foundation, Advanced and Speciality Course. The next 5 years saw a great deal of work go into this, but I continued to plough on in class working with each of the Reflexes in turn. Soon I was trying to bring it into my Vinyasa Yoga class as well, which was much more tricky but so beneficial that it was worth pursuing. And within 7 years, all my classes, workshops and festival workshops were all about the Reflexes.

Once we were confident that the Yoga for Autism material had been covered, and written about Yotism, we embarked on our very first 200-hour Reflex Yoga Teacher Training. Again, as it was a new course, and although we had a lot of intellectual and practical knowledge, it was still another step to work out how I could teach someone else to teach what I knew. And it bought an ever-deeper insight into how the Reflexes work. We now had 8 students who were about to launch into their very own Reflex Yoga Journey.

Many of their stories (with their permission of course) appear in the pages of this book, as we journey in our knowledge and understanding of what the Primitive Reflexes are and how they affect our body, with regards to the practice of yoga.

Firstly, though, I feel that we need to have a brief look at my background in yoga, as this also informs you how it is that Reflex Yoga has evolved.

I began my teacher training with the BWY (British Wheel of Yoga), which is a correspondence school of yoga. I did most of my work myself really. The material provided was very basic and was mainly interested in the postural aspect of yoga.

I believe I learnt as much from my Iyengar Yoga teacher, whose class I was attending religiously, week on week, at the local yoga centre. There wasn't much choice in 1997 as to styles of Yoga, especially in Reading, where I was living at the time, and we were in a dark, not too warm room, behind the swimming pool. I felt, however, as if it were a secret cave that only the few would enter. She was an excellent teacher, if rather dry, as is the way with Iyengar. But I loved her classes, and she taught me more than the BWY.

The BWY taught me the intellectual part of posture, breath and relaxation but the true learning happened in real-time. I remember cycling in the snow one November evening, wondering what on earth I was doing. But as I cycled back, I didn't even notice the cold, as I felt so good within myself. I did know I wanted more; on a more spiritual level, I felt very, very lost.

I qualified in early 1999 and began by teaching my friends. I did a 10-week course for free. I was rubbish – I could see that myself – but I knew that most of my learning had to happen in the act of teaching. I was then recruited to teach at the local leisure centre (these were the days when there were only 5 teachers in Reading, a town with a population of 30,000 – oh how times have changed!).

Many years before, when my eldest daughter was only 18 months old, my partner at the time had been convinced by one of his friends who had recently attended a Vipassana meditation course to attend one himself. I remember how the night before they left, they had all gone out to the pub and in the morning as they dragged themselves out of their hungover sleepiness all red-eyed and pale, they left for Herefordshire. A 3-hour drive. Ten days later, I opened the door to three very bright-eyed, alert and smiley people and the change in my partner was to be seen to be believed. For the next three months, he didn't drink, he meditated every morning, and we had one of the best times in our relationship.

The memory of this still lingered with me for a few months after we returned from Thailand, as now my daughter was old enough for me to leave her for 10 days. And though I had tried other forms of meditation, none of them had ever really affected me for very long.

Ten days seemed like such a long time – long enough to really find out what it was all about. Again, I had no idea what I was letting myself into. I asked a few questions and received even fewer answers, but I was still keen to go. So, in August 1999, the August of the solar eclipse – I remember it well as it happened right in the middle of my course – I found myself at Dhamma Dipa Meditation Centre in Pencoyd, Herefordshire, UK.

I have done many courses since, but I still remember this first one very clearly. I was sharing a room with 3 other young ladies about my age and there was little privacy and a lot of sleeping on my part. A bird had made its nest just outside our bedroom window and the fledglings chirruped a lot! The days rolled by, but by the 6th day, I was deep into meditation and had had many realisations and deep understandings, not to mention a few blissful moments!

The biggest surprise, however, was when I got back on the mat. My level of body awareness had gone perhaps from 5% to 95% and I could not believe how different my body felt and how much this changed how I taught. I couldn't believe how penetrating my mind was to be able to FEEL. And from this moment on, my practice became much more somatic – it was about awakening the connection between body and mind.

After my relationship broke down in 2002, I moved to London with a new partner. By this point, I had got heavily into meditation and had attended 2 courses and helped on 1. My new partner was also keen to find out what it was all about, and I attended my 3rd and 4th course this same year. I also began to teach and attend Ashtanga Yoga classes at the North London Buddhist Centre.

Ashtanga was a revelation to me. The dedication and discipline were something I knew I needed and even though Vipassana was teaching me mental discipline, Ashtanga began to teach me physical discipline.

The class was from 6.30 am to 9.30 am and you could arrive at any point and begin. There was a teacher on-site to monitor and help, if necessary, but the learning was purely by yourself. I had a book, so I knew which poses followed which and I worked hard, sweated a lot and relaxed beautifully at the end.

What I learnt most from Ashtanga however, apart from discipline, was that not all bodies were made equal and that forcing myself into something was not a good thing, no matter what the teacher told me. I had never had anyone take autonomy over my body and I was soon put off when one day the teacher stood on my hip to stretch it and hurt it badly. It didn't recover for weeks. This isn't an unusual story in Ashtanga Yoga and as my first experience under a lineage-based yoga approach, I was not impressed!

I continued to meditate and to attend courses over the next year and due to schooling issues, my partner and I decided to move to Herefordshire where there was a good Steiner school, and we were near the Vipassana Meditation Centre. More courses ensued, sometimes twice a year and then in the summer of 2007 another part of the yoga puzzle was put in place, as I met Jay Rossi of Kashmir Yoga in Nottingham.

Once again Santosa Yoga camp was the scene, a rainy one if I remember, and Jay was the star of the year. (There's always a star teacher – it's a totally organic thing, not planned – but there's always someone everyone flocks to because they are new and exciting.) Jay's classes were packed, and he taught in a way that spoke to me. Throughout the whole class, I can remember prodding Nicole and my partner and asking repeatedly, "Surely this guy has done a Vipassana Course?!" The way he spoke about the body was nothing short of hypnotising and you could feel that he was accessing a part of the mind whilst practising, that had hereto not been used. For me, he brought Vipassana and movement together to form meditation in motion. Imagine the shock when I asked after the class and found out that no, he had never attended a 10-day course! I was impressed enough to join his teacher training the following year and was not surprised to find 5 other people from Santosa Yoga Camp at his training too.

Training in Kashmir Yoga was eye-opening and a joy. So different to any other kind of training or workshop I had ever attended. Over a whole year, one Sunday a month we drove up from Herefordshire to Nottingham, and it was always a delight. Each lesson was a treasure trove of technique that was new to me and that spoke to me deeply. I learned many new things pertaining to embodiment, and somatic and the nervous system.

What I took with me into class was the idea that individuals respond differently to bodywork and that your vocal cueing must cater for everyone. This concept was new to me – having trained mainly in the old school yoga thus far, I was used to being the voice of wisdom, of knowing what was right for my students and never questioned the lineage that I had inherited.

This was the first time I began to wonder if the student actually had needs that I did not know about – that maybe they needed to explore their own bodies and make their own decisions. And that I was a vehicle for their discovery not the master of it.

Kashmir Yoga is based on the work of John Klein. His influence on yoga and a lot of other bodywork, is the idea that humans prefer certain senses: auditory, visual or kinetic. Appealing to these through your cues, helps others to come into their body in a way that speaks to them with ease. There were many techniques mixed in from other disciplines like Tai Chi and Chi Gong, as well as other bodywork techniques Klein had a hand in developing. Again, my yoga teaching changed for the better. I spent many years incorporating what I knew into my teaching and learning about how different approaches help one embody and breathe with ease.

It was this that I was teaching at Santosa Yoga Camp when the seeds of Reflex Yoga were sewn by the miraculous crawling transformation in my son.

What I hadn't considered initially, was the journey that I would personally go on to release my lifetime of accumulated trauma. As all humans, I was not a child who had gotten away without a lot of traumas in my body and mind. One of my earliest memories is a car accident I had in Peru. This I remembered in detail but hadn't realised how it was affecting my body. I had flown out of the car, hit my head on a bus and passed out. This single event affected my body at a young age and continued to do so until I finally released the trauma held in my body at the ripe age of 51.

Not long after, when I was 5, my mother left the country to move to the UK first. I didn't follow for another year. Moving to this country was a trauma. In Lima, I had been surrounded by many members of my family both adults and children. It was warm, and summer was all about the sea. The UK, in comparison, was cold and damp and it was a shock to my system. I remember in infant school crying and complaining to the teachers that they were cruel, making us go outside on such cold days. Darkness enveloped me early in the day. I was used to steady hours of sunrise at 6am, sunset at 6pm and I could not understand the language, sense of humour or rules of the world around me. I spent 6 months in a strange world of my mind, feeling very far from all humans and the planet I lived on.

As I grew, family life became difficult. It resulted in me being sent back to Peru at 11 to stay with my father and his new family (my sister was 2 and my brother yet to be born). I had to make another shift, as by this point, I had completely forgotten Spanish, the rules of this land and had to learn a whole new way of living. It was intense and again I found myself in this in-between land. I was lucky and the children at my new school were very keen to draw me in. This time, it didn't take so long. I was developing however, a sense of otherness, of not belonging anywhere, which I carried with me to adulthood. I could withdraw at the slightest difficulty socially and coming back from the abyss was always hard.

These two incidents are examples we can all find variations of, in different circumstances, in different times and continents yet we all know none of us pass through childhood without events, out of our control that affect us. Some of us really have much worse rides than others and the consequences can be life-limiting beyond belief. I was lucky, I had family to love and support me through – many don't.

My work in yoga initially helped me more than it helped my students. Yet as I became more mature in bodywork, meditation and life in general, my drive to help others has increased. Now that I have integrated most of the trauma I was carrying, I am keen to help anyone and everyone who is keen to heal. Most find me when they realise that talking therapy has reached its limit, and who instinctively know the body holds the key.

* * *

Reflex Yoga really is an extraordinary body of work that has the power to unblock blocks in an accessible and pleasant way. Blocks that you were perhaps so unconsciously holding, you didn't know were there. They hold you stuck in both body, mind and spirit. Reflex Yoga can help you to begin to release these blocks. This fusion of Yoga with neuroscience can enable change and give you a glimpse into how your body and your life could be. It facilitates an awareness of what is possible and opens you up to a better life. These forgotten healing reflex movements when integrated into yoga, and on their own, can transform your movement so you can really feel and move in new ways, however much other bodywork you have done previously. They can help bring a fuzzy mind into focus, help you be present. They can help you access your higher states of mind, connecting you to your inner self and ultimately your higher power, Spirit, God, Pachamama, whatever you choose to call her/him/they.

CHAPTER 1

Introduction to Reflexes

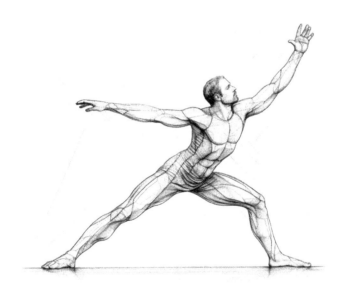

Our bodies are primed for survival. The destiny of every neurological impulse you have from the moment they are activated *in utero*, is to help you to survive. Our cells follow an order that step by step, small division by small division, transforms us from a mass of cells into functioning human beings, prepared to survive the first few months after birth. We learn to breastfeed, wean, sit, crawl, walk and be educated and grow into well-rounded adults. The miracle that is our growth *in utero* and beyond never ceases to amaze me.

This process is not smooth for most of us, as trauma, both mental and physical, both extreme and mild will influence how smooth and well-rounded we become. What is less known in this process is the role of the primitive reflexes and that they manage the entire process from tiny cell to adult human.

In this chapter, I will explain the role that the Primitive Reflex System has on our development, both physically, emotionally and spiritually and help you to understand why knowing this is important for our yoga practice.

It is almost miraculous that our first impulses of neurological development are done through movement and rhythm; yet deep down, we know it makes sense. Rhythm is seared into our systems, and we know it. Our Primitive Reflex System oversees making the movements happen automatically in our bodies when we are infants and beyond. Even though we are all wired differently, we all go through these same natural early stages of development and movement. How differently we may do these movements influences exactly how we function today, making each of us unique, even though we have all passed through the same neurological initiation.

There are unexpected influences that can interfere with this wiring-up process inside us, and children and adults alike may experience a difference or interruption in their nervous system as a result. The latest neurological research can now help us understand what is happening when the system is not set up properly. With Reflex Integration work, we can learn how to undo some of these patterns that form without our control when so young. We can create new movement patterns in our bodies and open the pathways to new learning.

Yoga brings us back home to ourselves; we begin to land in our body and are free from our mind and ego. Through body movement and breathwork techniques, we strengthen and reorganise our body, mind and our sense of self from the inside out. We can also change our neurological patterns. We have either experienced this ourselves, or seen others change over time, through some sort of physical activity. Our body looks and feels different, and we have new insights and healing. Often a new direction in life has also been embarked upon.

Primitive Reflex Integration and yoga make very good bed fellows. One can see clearly how the two modalities of working with the body and nervous system function can be brought together to work together. As I am a yoga teacher, most of this book uses yoga as an example of how you can integrate the reflexes in the body. Yet yoga is not the only modality out there. I am sure other types of bodywork would benefit greatly from having this work added to it.

Depending on the type of yoga you are doing or how you are personally doing it, it is not always the case that yoga is helping change your neurology for the better. Some types of yoga cause you more stress! If Primitive Reflex Systems have not been released, when the body or mind is under considerable stress, the body will automatically 'reflex' into old survival patterns. So, you could be practising yoga without realising that these reflexes are holding you in patterns that are not helpful but are so familiar to you, they feel normal. This explains why some people still need to return to the osteopath after they have been practising yoga for many years and perhaps give up yoga because it makes them 'worse'. No amount of stretching seems to help release these patterns; you need to use Primitive Reflex Integration exercises to do so. These integration exercises help to set up the body for better functional movement that may have been forgotten due to small or large traumas to your body. Primitive Reflex work helps you to release the holding patterns that may be working against you to help you to stretch or move in a healthier way.

Reflex Yoga goes back to these primal movements – these movements that in infancy, would have released and integrated the Reflexes naturally. With consistent practice, these movements help any Reflexes still retained, to release and integrate now. It also heals the system and forms new building blocks in the physical, developmental and emotional pathways for the rehabilitation of the body and mind.

Those that have practised Reflex Yoga have reported that the awareness of their bodies increases dramatically. All over body awareness can be achieved. If there are any tensions in the body, these are immediately obvious and what's more, there is now the ability to relax these areas at will and so perform asanas in a safe and relaxed manner.

If there are chronic holding patterns, then these are also eased. For example, someone with a frozen shoulder will begin to understand how they are exacerbating the problem by holding tension in the shoulder (Moro Reflex, Asymmetric Tonic Neck Reflex – ATNR) and even when in pain, can begin to feel the 'anger' being taken out of the shoulder. If someone has very tight hamstrings (Fear Paralysis Reflex – FPR) and cannot forward bend, they will notice how they are drawing their legs in towards the body rather than letting them go into the ground. Once they have realised this, they will then be able to relax them, and so hamstrings will become elastic once more. When talking with someone who is experiencing chronic pain, they will always describe a holding pattern they feel unable to let go of. It is involuntary, a 'reflex' that needs to remember how to let go.

If there is a persistent holding pattern, then this will begin to be released. For example, a student who consistently does Downward Dog in a crooked way (Spinal Galant Reflex) will begin to feel that they are crooked, whereas before they thought they were pushing through the hands and body in a consistent manner and that their hips were level. They will begin to feel the weaker side and even out the inconsistency, pushing and strengthening the weaker side until they are straight again. They will naturally level out their hips without too much effort as the new pattern will feel normal.

Others will begin to see how they are compensating with tension when one part of them is weak. For example, someone who is doing a Half Scorpion pose, will feel the tension in the back of their neck (Tonic Labyrinthic Neck Reflex – TLR) and will be able to relax this tension at will. Another student who has weak core muscles will have tension in the shoulder stand (TLR) and will learn to isolate the head and so use their core muscles more distinctly.

These are examples of the raised awareness we learn as we begin to integrate our reflexes into our bodies. I often say that this is the first step in Reflex Yoga, understanding that we are holding tension, we are crooked or weak on one-sided. Or it may be much more subtle than that, but awareness begins to build up and you are able to feel at this more subtle level. A yoga teacher may be able to point something out to you that isn't quite straight or right, but could you feel it? Was your own awareness picking up on these subtleties? And how would you remember not to repeat, what is in essence, a habit pattern of your body?

The first mission of Reflex Yoga is to begin by having you, the student, notice these patterns yourself, tune into them and then know what to do about them to release them.

The second mission of Reflex Yoga is to help you to understand how being better connected to your body can also make you better connected neurologically. This gives us access to better brain function, more emotional stability, better focus and spiritual connection, amongst many other benefits.

The mind-body connection is well known in yoga, but we rarely look at it from the point of view of neurology. As you will see, many parts of our brain are involved in emotional intelligence, understanding and development. What is vital to understand from the offset, is that if an individual is living in survival mode most of the time, under duress and stress, they will not have access to the neural connections for the emotional regulation centres of the brain. Like the hidden disability that it is, mental health issues will abound when in perpetual survival mode and the individual will not have any way of changing this until they successfully come out of survival mode.

Reflex Yoga not only helps you to come out of your survival patterns, but it also gives you better brain connections. This allows you to access the emotional (limbic) parts of the brain, making new connections, or the ones you already have more efficient and stable. In turn, this gives people with mental health issues hope. Now here is a set of easy movements, that can help put me in a better state of mind, every day, not just after yoga class. What's more, these movements take minutes to do and are easily achievable daily. The empowerment this gives an individual is priceless.

The third mission of Reflex Yoga is to allow those of us who are functioning in survival mode access to our higher thinking centre (prefrontal cortex) where our sense of Spirituality is. Again, when we are constantly concerned with survival and under excess stress, we cannot also be concerned with the larger questions about our existence. We are too busy surviving.

This can mean that all the spiritual practices that we are attempting are helping us, but we aren't accessing them in quite the depth we think. We don't become aware of this until we are out of survival mode, when everything makes sense again in a much different way.

Personally, I have worked with body awareness practices for over 20 years. I have worked with my mind, meditating for just as long. All the while, I have been aware of others' spiritual practices and attempted to have my own. It was only after I came out of my own trauma and survival mode that I felt a coming together of all these three practices into one whole moment. In that moment, I am present in my body, mind and spirit simultaneously. I inhabit the fullness that is the self in harmony and equanimity. It was only after having this experience that I realised that I had lived most of my life 'blown apart' by my trauma. I was blind to it until then.

In this state of wholeness, I was truly able to begin to understand my role in life, my connection to the Divine and how I was moving in the world.

It was Reflex Yoga that helped teach my body and mind how to come out of trauma and stay there. Creating new patterns in the body where I was not constantly scanning the environment for danger and being always prepared to run or fight, opened the door for me to become my true whole, settled self. My hope for you is that through this book, you will achieve this too.

NEURAL DEVELOPMENT

Neurodevelopment starts with movement. Movement is essential for healthy brain and nervous system development. We need movement to grow, control our bodies, process our environment and ultimately reach spiritual freedom.

When our pathways of movement are not fed the correct input, we do not develop our senses fully or efficiently. This affects our levels of body awareness, our emotional equanimity, our ability to learn, focus and reach and stretch ourselves into a more wholesome existence.

When we are stuck in primitive brain functioning, or back brain hijacking, we are in survival mode most of the time. As this is an automatic brain function or reflex, we can find it difficult, if not impossible, to come out of it without the right kind of physical input. The kind of physical input we had *in utero* and as infants.

At birth, the neural connections between the different areas of the brain are minimal. An infant's brain needs healthy myelination to make the smooth connections it needs to develop fully. Myelination happens through repetitive movements in the body. Myelination is the process of lubricating the axon and acts as a lubricant for nerve fibres to be able to travel and make the first connections in the brain. Myelin is made up of fatty lipids and proteins that accumulate around the neurons, and they play an essential role in the health and function of nerve cells, the brain and the nervous system. The reason brain matter looks white is because of the numerous amounts of myelinated brain cells. The myelination process is vitally important to healthy central nervous system functioning. Myelination begins *in utero* when a foetus is about 16 weeks and is happening in the brain throughout adulthood.

A good visual way to understand myelination is to think of a neural pathway as a long tube, down which we would like our information (a ball in this example) to travel. If there are numerous exit holes the ball could fall out of, or there are kinks and turns the ball could get stuck around, then information may be slow or never arrive. With myelination, the tube is surrounded by a fatty greasy lubricant that allows the ball to move swiftly and without distractions or deviation.

Another way to visualise the process of myelination is to think of the brain as a map of a country with millions of tiny cart tracks taking messages to different parts of the country. At birth, these cart tracks are not particularly effective, and the messages are passed all over the brain without much direction. As time (and movements) take us through our involuntary primitive reflex movements, we begin to make certain roads more important and through a pruning process will eventually finish with an efficient transport system including many motorways (myelin pathways).

Think of a baby learning to use a spoon for the first time. To begin with, the pathway to the mouth is not known and most of the food finishes up on the floor and all over the table. With practice and repetition, we will eventually work out the pathway to our mouth and for a time it will be pretty hit and miss as to whether the food reaches our stomach. However, we keep on repeating these moves and eventually, we are consistent with this pathway. By the time we have myelinated this pathway, our conscious awareness falls away, and as an adult, we are barely aware of the spoon as we lift it to our lips and converse while we eat.

This pathway is like a motorway from London to Edinburgh. Once we embark on the journey, we know the message is on its way and we can sit back and relax, knowing that our end destination is assured. When we have trauma, or back brain hijacking or any kind of neurological difference, this smooth messaging may be disturbed. We may find ourselves travelling to Liverpool and then Glasgow before we arrive in Edinburgh making the journey longer, more tiring and leaving us much more frazzled. This helps us understand why for someone on the spectrum or with ADHD for example, some tasks seem to be so difficult and exhausting.

Our early development is centred around our sensory perception. This sensory stimulus helps us make sense of our environment and our experiences. This portal into the world lets us know what is happening around us and provide us with information as to what is happening inside of us, so we can respond effectively. This information also helps us to understand why it is that when we are under stress or have a neurodiversity, the sensory system can be overwhelmed, and we can be triggered even further into stress.

PRIMITIVE REFLEXES AND MOVEMENT

Rhythmical movements improve the myelination process which is why we call this style of yoga neurodevelopmental and why it is so powerful at making physiological changes. Hence the more opportunities we are given to practice these movements, the better wired-up we can become, and the more lubricated certain connections become. These effective movements create the right type of muscle tone and connectivity which in the first stages of life are all about head, neck and trunk mastery and control.

It has been estimated that every minute in the life of a newborn, 4.7 million new nerve cell branches are created. This maturing brain will continue to develop throughout childhood. However, it is the first year and the integration of the Primitive Reflex System that lays down the foundation for later development. Brain development does not happen by itself, it needs the right kind of stimulation from the body and the sensory system.

The brain becomes flooded when the survival system is permanently switched on and we find ourselves in fight or flight most of the time. Then the sympathetic nervous system is functioning all the time, and the process of pruning is not successfully achieved. Pruning is a process that is highly important. It is a key part of development because it eliminates the connections that are not used often enough, which provides room for the most important networks of connections to grow and expand.

THE INITIAL NEURODEVELOPMENTAL JOURNEY

At 5 weeks of gestation *in utero*, the intrauterine reflexes emerge, leading at around 9 weeks to the first of the Primitive Reflexes. This growth continues throughout foetal stages at about a rate of 250,000 neurons every second, until it is estimated that we are born with 86 billion neurons.

After birth, the number of neurons does not increase in most areas of the brain. However, through neurogenesis, there are some areas of the brain where new neurons are added. The hippocampus is the only part of the brain that continues to generate new neurons throughout life. It is the basis for long term memory, spatial awareness and our survival responses like 'Fight, Flight or Fright'.

At birth, the brain is about 25% of the size it will be as an adult and by the age of two it is about 80%. It takes many years to develop all the connections necessary to be able to control impulses, organise information, plan and problem solve. Therefore, the harder we work as a baby, the less hard we work throughout life. Movement and sensory stimulation are essential for healthy connections for synaptic growth and neurogenesis (neural creation).

The Reflex System is the kick-starter on this journey of development that enables movement, growth and pathways to independence.

A timeline for brain pruning follows these times loosely:

Around 6 weeks, when the baby starts to gain visual focus.

Around 1 year, when the infant starts to make the physical connections for walking.

Around 2 years, when a toddler starts making the connections for language.

Around 6 years, when a child cognitively develops reading and writing skills.

Around 16 years, at the time of prefrontal growth and executive functioning – (problem-solving skills, decision making, judgement, impulse control, emotional reasoning).

Around 21 years, at the time of greater cognitive and emotional growth, with skills in academia, independence and the formation of solid friendships/relationships.

Brain growth and plasticity allow for great variation in and beyond these 'critical periods.' Neural branching and pruning are ongoing throughout life. If we engage in varied life experiences, the brain will respond, using established connections and growth.

BRAIN STRUCTURES

Understanding the brain is obviously a fascinating topic. Neuroscientists and lay people in this modern age are finding out more and more about its abilities, capacity and structure.

We once believed that there was a certain age beyond which you supposedly would not produce any more new brain cells. This has now been found to be untrue. The knowledge about brain plasticity is still in its infancy, especially for those with an injury, but more and more research is added every year.

The brain develops from the bottom up, with three main parts: the hindbrain, midbrain and forebrain.

As an infant it is our hindbrain that is in control. This is where the correct connecting up of Primitive Reflexes originates for overall development. As the brain grows, with the right primal survival mechanisms in place and making more connections, the forebrain begins to take over control.

The brainstem is the home of our Primitive Reflexes. When the Primitive Reflexes do not integrate efficiently, neural maturation can stay delayed, and the brainstem can still be controlling some of your movements, making them stiff or jerky.

The only part of the brain that is fully matured at birth is the brainstem. It is responsible for survival e.g. breathing, heartbeat and digestion. These are all reflexive movements and autonomic functions of the nervous system. When an infant matures, the brainstem should gradually let go of the need to control some of these movements. The baby starts to gain its own control over its own body in order to become upright, for example. The brain then starts to take control from the higher levels of brain function.

If the brain stem continues to control brain function due to foetal or maternal stress for example, then the Primitive Reflex System will not get the stimulation it needs to integrate fully, and these reflexes will stay active. Staying active, we will feel unsafe and be perpetually in survival mode. This will have knock on effects on our development including postural control, emotional maturity, impulse control, academic learning, comprehension and movement patterns.

Scientific research has proven that yoga and meditation have targeted positive effects on the diencephalon and the forebrain. It specifically thickens the wall of the neocortex, enlarges the amygdala and lights up the hippocampus.

A fusion of yoga and Primitive Reflex Integration is powerful in changing developmental brain chemistry and making new connections.

Rhythmic movements at any stage of life can be used to strengthen neural pathways and integrate the brain.

CASE STUDY

In my years of teaching Baby Yoga, I have seen how a traumatic birth can affect a young baby's ability to breastfeed, settle and sleep. I have talked to mothers who are struggling to work out what can make their baby happy. I have then shown them a few Reflex moves to do together which have helped enormously to settle their baby. As mentioned in my Introduction, Baby Yoga is where this method was first trialled.

Baby A is displaying a sitting position which is slouched. Watching a baby trying to sit in this way, you can visibly see how much hard work it is, and it is not surprising that the baby prefers to be lying down more than sitting. This slouching sitting position is unusual as most babies have a way of sitting upright so naturally and without effort (thanks to the Symbiotic Tonic Neck Reflex – STNR). It is rare to see a baby sit this way, so in class it was obvious to me that something was up with their nervous system.

The mother did not attend many Baby Yoga sessions as she came late to classes (when the baby was already 6 months) and returned to work 3 months later. As the class was a general class and it is not ethical to diagnose or give unsolicited advice, I barely mentioned the issue to the mother but asked her to contact me in the future if she ever needed help with her son in any way.

Five years later, Mum called me for some help, as her child had now been formally diagnosed with Autism. A little late, we got to work....

More recently, working with older children in a nursery, I spied a baby slouch sitting through the window of the door of the room I work in. Having a couple of minutes spare, I asked if I could come in and show her carers a few movements that would help her. After a very brief demonstration, I put the baby on the floor as the staff 'oohed' and 'aahed.' She was now sitting bolt upright. It lasted only half a minute, as the pattern is new, but straight away it was rectified. The staff are now, not only aware of the help movements give, but also of their importance. I have watched this baby for a few months and her posture is now normal. She only needed to be shown the correct movements for her brain to fine tune what was ready to mature and now it does it naturally. The younger the child, the easier it is to help them.

CONCLUSION

As mentioned at the beginning of this chapter, we now know how movement and neurodevelopment go hand in hand. We learnt that movement forms the basis of our brain hook up and how different parts of our brain come online at different times. We know how we can reinforce certain pathways and prune others, and how all of this is done through a natural process called Primitive Reflex Integration.

We know from our own practice that yoga is transformational and now we can understand how the movement we pursue in yoga; along with breathwork, (more of that later) changes us from the inside out.

We are beginning to understand why the movements practised in Reflex Yoga are even more transformational and together with the practice of yoga, we can now begin to imagine what a healing tool we have on our hands.

CHAPTER 2

Foot Hand Face Reflex

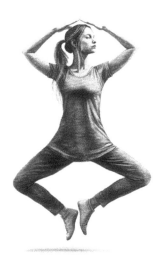

We start with these three Reflexes for a reason. As you will see, they are the foundation of healthy development in infanthood and give stability to the work that we do later. It is important that we feel safe and relaxed as we begin to teach our nervous system new patterns. For some of us, these patterns are so new, that they can scramble our system if we are not careful and do not follow the correct order of integration. We advise that you follow the sequence of integration exactly as it is laid out in this book, tempting though it may be to skip ahead to what we think we need.

Our nervous system has the capability of building new neurological pathways, and these pathways need to have good foundations. Feet, Hand and Face (FHF) Reflexes are some of the most intricate, yet important pathways that we build these foundations on. For this reason, we dedicate much time to them at the beginning of our work with anyone, including ourselves. Without the FHF Reflexes, our whole system is out of whack, meaning all the other reflexes that integrate afterwards (Survival Reflexes, Postural Reflexes, Transitional Reflexes, etc) may also be out of whack too.

With the example of the baby in the last chapter, I recognised what further integration she would need for her postural reflexes. I would have started with the Feet Hands and Face, as even a baby would have felt out of sorts, not remembering my session with me kindly if I hadn't. We will also see the importance of bonding in this chapter. In fact, often when I go and pick up children from their classroom, the young ones look at me happily and say, "Round and round the garden?" The children's song I sing when I massage their hands. The rhyme 'Round and round the garden,' is a great bonding song I use when I massage their hands. Their memory of me goes straight to the feelings of safety and bonding, that the hand reflexes give. The other, harder work is completely forgotten.

Here there are three Reflexes bunched together, to integrate together, that also have the capacity to integrate separately. They are integrating at the same time on the developmental arc. They work together to achieve the one type of result, but separately to achieve another. Working together, they stabilise the nervous system and help the other Reflexes develop smoothly. We will have a look at each Reflex independently of each other and then see how extraordinary they are when we work them together.

The support structure of the Feet, Hand and Face Reflexes are like the box around a Jenga game. It helps neaten, line up and support the building blocks of development. They provide stability. Without them, your Jenga stack would be wonky and the Reflexes in your system may not have integrated as well as they could have. As more blocks are added over time, they continue to provide support.

If you have ever watched a young baby when exploring new impressions of the world around them, they are often flapping their hands or kicking their feet in excitement. It helps them to emotionally organise themselves with either excitement or frustration. Babies will extend their hands and put things in their mouths and learn about the world through their feet, hands and mouth. I'm sure, if some of us start watching ourselves, we will find that when you are concentrating hard, you may be twiddling something with your hands, tapping your foot or perhaps making faces with your mouth, even biting your lips.

These reflexes are important in yoga and all movement practices for us to integrate a sense of where the end of our limbs are in space (proprioception) and feelings of safety within the body. The information we receive about where we are in space and how safe our environment is will help us to start the process of relaxing. Can you imagine what it would feel like if you were unable to feel your feet? How ungrounded you would be, how you would be floating all the time?

What if your hands were not well connected to you, how tiring would it feel to thread a needle? Would you do well in school if it was a struggle to use your hands? What would your handwriting be like if your hands were always too tense or too slack? In yoga, we may find that some poses are too hard for our hands as they are so tightly held, or that we are hypermobile in our hands and find it impossible to hold hand poses for long.

Now what would happen, if every morning you woke up with a sore jaw because you've been grinding your teeth all night long? What condition would your teeth be in? And how would you relax at the end of a yoga class if you'd spent the entirety of it clenching your jaw? Looking deeper into each of these three Reflexes and how they work together as a whole will enormously help in our yoga practice.

When we can maintain an awareness both conscious and unconscious in our body, of our feet, hands and face then we will find movement in yoga, even in more complex poses and deeper mindful exercises much more fluid and safer. We may feel able to explore something which is new to us with confidence and calm.

There is not only development in the physical realm when we practice yoga but also in the emotional/spiritual realm. Development isn't all just about the body. As neuroscience has proven, the brain is 80% concerned with what is happening in the body. This means our experience of life is mainly coming from our body feedback so when this changes, so will our experience of ourselves in the world.

When we are fully integrated in our hand, feet and mouth Reflexes, we experience the world from a place of connection and belonging. We are fully in this world, bonded to it and to those who inhabit it with us. We can pull in and grasp from this world everything we feel we may need; from practical things like earning a living, to more esoteric aspects like trusting the Universe has our back. We can hold ourselves, be integrated into our sense of self and bonded with the emotional person inside of us, our inner being. We can practice true self-care not just giving ourselves the occasional luxury bath, for example. We take care of ourselves understanding that in doing so we also take care of those around us. These concepts, though familiar in theory, become actualised as we live them day to day. It starts to feel natural to take care of ourselves first.

Belonging to ourselves is a concept that took me years to understand, let alone embody. It is a journey that I am still on. What I can say about this journey so far is that it has taken me from co-dependency and an anxious attachment style to an independent and connected woman. Connected with healthy boundaries, able to hold relationships on my own terms. Alone but not lonely.

Until I worked on these Reflexes, I had not realised that I clenched my hands when I was stressed, sometimes to the point of my thumb joint hurting. I also nearly always had my hands in a slightly closed position when my hands were at rest. I had also not realised how disconnected to my feet I really was. I mean, I could feel them, however, especially in times of stress, I seemed to cut them out of my body. Sometimes I would miss step, or worse. When I was learning to Snow Board and I was terrified, I twisted my ankle because I had not realised my boot was not strapped on properly, for example. Who has not accidently kicked a bookcase that has been in the same position for years in the middle of the night on the way to the loo? Me. I also knew that I clenched my jaw and ground my teeth in my sleep but what I had not realised was that this was contributing towards neck tension, and particularly a reoccurring frozen shoulder.

Much later in my journey, when I was working out the final tension of my held Moro Reflex, this would be the final piece of a jigsaw to rid me of shoulder tension forever. Underlying all my bravado, as a woman living in the modern world, and having had a few scary near misses with strange men in alleyways, I never really felt safe in the world. I would make myself walk in the dark, but I was always on alert. I would go to bed happily in an empty house, but I would secure my bedroom door. I much preferred to have someone else nearby. I remember the first time I slept alone in my detached house; we were so rural that we hardly ever locked the door. That night, I did. I knew I wouldn't settle without that extra security. These days, I couldn't tell you if the door is locked or not.

SELF-PRACTICE

We believe that the best way to learn about Reflexes is to experience them in our body ourselves and so understand their subtle and intrinsic nature. There are special links within this book you can use to access yoga videos so you can try out the technique for yourself.

Please feel free to visit **www.the-empowered-feminine.co.uk** for a hand-based yoga practice example. At the end of this book, there are details of how to access the videos that accompany this book, at:

www.the-empowered-feminine.co.uk

And afterwards, try and answer these questions for yourself:

How aware of your hands/feet/jaw were you, to begin with? Did this improve throughout the practice? How did this make you feel as you practised?

How did your body feel after the practice? How was your mind (more settled, more relaxed, a little phased out?) What was the overall quality of your sense of self? How do you feel now, after the practice has finished?

These Reflexes are vital for whole-body development:

Foot Reflexes: Once we have begun to integrate the Foot Reflexes, we will feel more stable on our feet and find ourselves more grounded and held securely in the space we inhabit. We start forming the foundations of where we are in our body and start to feel secure in this presence.

Hand Reflexes: When our hands have integrated their Reflexes, we are able to handle tasks with ease. We can master fine motor skills and form the bonds with our outside world. We can tackle the task of self-management, practical survival and creativity. The hands help us to feel and 'do' our way through life with greater ease.

Mouth Reflexes: When our Mouth Reflexes have integrated, we can organise sensory information, develop speech and language and form good attachments in the world. We can digest our world, support our learning and relax more in the security of being held and loved in the world.

Put together, these three Reflex areas are essential for whole body and brain development. They form part of our processing system, our postural management and the ability to support the whole self. In old age, these Reflexes can become stuck and if there is an overload of stress, adults can often feel the hands clench, the jaw lock or the toes curl in their shoes.

We have specific movements for these Reflexes to help to integrate them. They allow them to stay healthy and happy throughout the challenges of life. When an adult experiences these Reflexes as either retained or overactive, we can experience all sorts of symptoms such as bad posture, fatigue, heightened anxiety and addictive tendencies for example. These Reflexes are intrinsically connected to our nervous system response of fight, flight and fright.

In all of us, these Reflexes can be activated when we are in a trauma response, mild or strong. What is important to understand with these Reflexes, whether you have them mildly or with any strength, is that you can perhaps have a feeling of being unsafe or disassociated from your own body because of your nervous system not being stable. We will find our nervous system so happy to jump from one state to another without any warning and so we will find ourselves hyper-alert for the next possible change ahead.

These 3 Reflexes are also a neural stabiliser. The better integrated these Reflexes are, the less nervous the nervous system is likely to spin off into a primitive reaction/reflex. We are more likely to remain stable under stress and in moments of trauma. Have you ever felt yourself sink into a chair or sofa, once the danger is over? Coming back into your body through the Feet, Hands or Face or all of these, is a quick way to achieve the same result.

Safety isn't something that we can think ourselves into. When we feel unsafe, no amount of verbal reassurance will do. We cannot cognise safety. We need to feel it: feel it in our bodies and so these Reflexes go a long way to making our bodies feel safe.

INTEGRATING FEET, HANDS AND FACE REFLEX

The feet: The Babinski and Plantar Reflexes

Without a sense of our feet, the body-brain will be impacted by lack of Foot Integration. There could be feelings of not being grounded, of flitting/flying purposeless through life. Of not knowing what we are here on this earth to do. There may be direction but not quite being able to access how to get there. What steps to take to achieve it? In more stressful moments, the feeling of disembodiment and being overwhelmed or ungrounded sensations can lead us to make rash decisions which don't really make sense later, or simply to shut off completely from life.

To be in your feet is to land home in your body. To have presence in your sense of self, even to be able to connect to your inner being with ease and have a knowing that we are not alone, we can tune into the sense of our 'mother' who is always there for us. Feeling the earth beneath our feet brings us closer to nature, to the terrain we are travelling on and our connection to the magic of life increases. Life no longer is just about what goes on in our heads, what we think about. Life is all around us and we are as much part of it as the birds on the bird feeder in front of me as I write, right now.

There are two main Foot Reflexes, the Plantar Reflex and the Babinski Foot Reflex.

THE PLANTAR REFLEX

A way of checking for this Reflex in the feet is to apply pressure to the ball of the foot and see how much the toes curl in. If a child or adult experiences strong foot withdrawal or sensitivity, is it likely this Reflex is still active. An active Reflex can hinder walking, make our balance centre skewed and we can appear clumsy. Being upright is hard as the toes curl in. If it is overactive, we see tiptoe walking, feelings of instability and a constant state of fight or flight. This can lead to a dislike of change and rigid habits, lifestyle management, a need to control the environment and lack of concentration.

When the Plantar Reflex is active, we experience tight hamstrings, misaligned pelvis and a sense of falling forwards. We have a sense of being in perpetual movement, finding stillness difficult, especially when standing up. This leads to feelings of overwhelm, falling short of the mark and finding it hard to relax.

This Reflex starts to emerge *in utero* at around 12 weeks, is present at birth and should be integrated by around 8 months. It is thought to be a legacy of an earlier evolutionary stage of development where clinging was important. It is closely connected to the Central Nervous System (CNS).

BABINSKI FOOT REFLEX

To check for this Reflex, tickle the sole of the foot, if the toes curl out strongly, this reflex is present. When this Reflex is active, we have a sense of being in perpetual movement, finding stillness difficult, especially when standing up. This leads to feelings of overwhelm, falling short of the mark and finding it hard to relax.

This Reflex is present at the same time as the Plantar Reflex and is thought to be preparing the foot for weight baring (preparing for when the baby is learning to walk) and should be finishing integrating once we are standing up. It also has a part to play in helping us place our foot squarely on solid ground.

MOVEMENTS TO INTEGRATE THE PLANTAR REFLEX

Here follow some simple exercises for Feet Reflex Integration:

Tiptoes and Heels

Start with lifting the toes off the floor and place them back down. Then the heels off the floor and place them back down. Then start to rock between the two, tiptoes and heels, tiptoes and heels. Don't worry about getting high on your tiptoes or rocking far back on the heels. Try instead to keep a gentle rhythm going where you can relax, as if you were on a rocking chair. Keep this up until you feel a change in the body. It could be a tiredness in the halves, shins or feet. It could be a new sensation elsewhere in the body or it could be a thought pattern that comes in from nowhere, a frustration, fatigue or worry about something. These are all signs that the nervous system has had enough for now. Take a breath and, as if the out-breath were rain, let it trickle down to your feet and water your new roots.

Barefoot Walking

On a warm day, take off your shoes and walk outside, noticing all the different surfaces, textures and temperatures of the grass, stone, mud, etc you walk on.

Fun Walking

Walk on the outsides of bare feet. Bend your knees and put the weight on the outsides of your feet. Walk up and down your matt or around the room.

Now walk on the inside of your feet, knees knocked together a bit; put the weight on the big toes and inner arches. Walk up and down your matt or around the room. Next walk on tiptoes around the room and finally walk on your heels. Have a moment now to stand on the whole foot. Feel into the sensation of having the whole foot on the floor, really tune into the weight distribution. Take a breath, and as if the out-breath were rain, let it trickle down to your feet and water your new roots.

Spiky Ball Massage

If you have a soft spiky ball and your feet can tolerate it, run a spiky ball up and down the feet, along the ball, bridge and over your toes. Repeat a few times, if it feels okay to do so. If it feels too much, try a firm spikey ball instead. If this is still too much, try giving yourself a firm foot massage first.

Foot Massage

Hold the foot in your hand and with both the thumbs run them up the centre of the sole of the foot and down and around the outside a few times. You can also use a fist and push your knuckles into the ball and heel of your foot. Massage the outer edges of your heels and gently pinch each toe. Try to massage the area at the top of the foot where it meets the toe joints.

Case Study

One of the children I have been working with at a nursery, let's call him Richard, had severe retained Plantar and Babinski Foot Reflexes. When I first met him, he was in a classroom of 30 children, pacing up and down a track of balance beams he had made for himself on his tiptoes! He kept falling over, but of course he had built this track to keep himself centred, as the noise in the room was so loud. I asked the staff if he did this regularly and they said it was all he ever did! Richard did not speak at all, only low hummed and he only ever looked at the floor.

I spent many weeks working on his Foot Reflexes. At first, it was all I could do to take off his shoes. Over many months we progressed, and he was then able to take his socks off and take all kinds of integration work for his feet. His favourite was to sit in the chair, relax and let me massage his feet. He would close his eyes and I could feel his whole body melt. He often wanted this at the beginning of our sessions, however, I'd keep the best till last!

What was astonishing is that within two weeks, he stopped pacing, building tracks and started to do other things within the room allocated to him. Still very much in his own world, he was now open to new input. Later on, I will mention Richard again as he begins to develop speech, eye contact and enters the world.

FOOT REFLEXES AND
YOGA PRACTICE

Maybe you are not well connected in your feet, and you often kick things by accident or misstep, or feel ungrounded a lot of the time. In yoga, we often mention the feet and talk about 'grounding' and 'rooting' the feet into the floor but perhaps some of us are unable to attain this, or even know what it feels like or what the yoga teacher means. This is where the Feet Integration exercises above will really help to increase your awareness of your feet and then you will all be starting from the same point of reference.

Within any yoga class that I hold, there is always a little footwork done first to help us all start from this same awareness and for us to feel safe in the new environment of the class. It takes longer for some than for others, but slowly over time, we will be able to access our sense of 'feet' far more swiftly as our nervous system integrates this pathway. We will begin to feel present within our bodies and within our yoga room environment. I often like this initial moment where you can visibly see students go from being in their heads to being in their bodies.

An example of how this can be used in a practice session – after some integration exercises, let's say 'Tiptoes and Heels,' is to continually bring your attention to your feet in every yoga pose that you do. See if you can discern how movement affects your weight distribution, how your toes move (or don't move) or how your arch reacts. You could recall the grounding effects of the integration exercises, reminding yourself continuously of how you felt immediately after an exercise and remembering how the feet sank into the ground and how the legs were able to sink into the floor with ease. You could practice some balancing exercises and compare how each foot feels after it has been stood on for a while. There are numerous ways to bring mindful movement and foot awareness together as the following examples demonstrate.

YOGA POSES FOR FOOTWORK:

Examples of good poses in yoga that work for this technique are:

Standing Forward Bends

Downward Dog

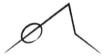

Triangle Forward Bends

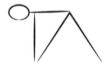

OTHER EXERCISES TO INTEGRATE FOOT REFLEXES

Raising Foot Awareness: Trace your feet

Standing on your feet. Bring your attention to the top of your right big toe. In your mind's eye, start to draw a line down the big toe towards the joint with your next other toe and up your second first toe to the tip. Keep drawing around your second toe, third toe, fourth toe and little toe. Continue to draw, down the outer edge of your foot, around the ankle and up the arch of your foot towards the tip of your big toe, where you started. Notice how you can feel the whole of your right foot on the floor and feel the difference between your right foot and your left foot.

Now take your attention to your left big toe. Once again begin to draw around the big toe, second toe, third toe, fourth toe and little toe. Bring your attention down the outer edge of your left foot, around the ankle and up the arch of your foot to meet the point where you started at the big toe. Notice the whole of your left foot on the floor. Feel every detail.

Now bring your awareness to both feet on the floor. Notice your weight distribution. Is your weight evenly distributed? Or are you more on the balls or on the heels? Are you leaning to the left or to the right? Bring your awareness to your feet and lean slightly forward and then slightly back. Do this a few times and then find the place where you are neither forward nor back but right in the middle. Now lean your weight a little left, then a little right. Move the weight side to side for a few moments and then find the place where you are neither left nor right, but right in the middle. Now circle your weight from right, then forward, then left then back. Do a few circles like this in both directions; and then, as you do your final circles, find the exact centre point.

How does it feel to be centred and grounded like this through your feet? What kind of feeling does it bring up?

Affirmations for Footwork:

"I stand strong and long and stable."
"I move in all directions with ease."

"My feet are grounded like the roots of a tree."

"I stand proud and stand my ground."

"I am here. I am present in my body."

"I have landed."

Other bodywork techniques that work for Footwork are:

- Tai Chi
- Chi Gong
- Martial Arts
- Climbing
- Walking and running

THE HAND REFLEXES

Hand Reflexes are a vital part of our neurological system, as they give us a more detailed and nourishing knowledge of our surroundings than our feet. With our hands, we explore the world and learn a lot from it, feeling like we know it and being able to bond to it. We form healthy human attachments, initially to our mother, then to our social group, to our partner in life and ultimately leading to having a sense of self, our inner being.

Without Hand Reflex Integration, we do not develop an understanding of love, of the rules of relationship and healthy touch. The social world is beyond our reach and communication is difficult, making play and fun hard to access. We may experience a lot of struggles mentally, as our mind pushes and pulls our understanding of these aspects of human nature, rather than being able to live with an innate knowledge of them.

Without our Hand Reflexes, we do not have a sense of the world and ourselves in it. Babies learn about the world by grasping, bringing things to their mouths, and so understanding, gaining knowledge of what the world is made of and therefore their role within it. Without this, we can walk through a room, our own living space and not be a part of it. It's there but we may not see it, sense it or feel ourselves in it. In more extreme cases, a human being that lives in your space would be unseen, part of the furniture so to speak, and may not be acknowledged at all. You may know they are there in a vague way, however you don't feel connected enough to them to even greet them.

When we have healthy Hand Integration, we can grasp towards us our most basic needs for survival. Work, shelter, cleanliness and food. However, we can also bring ourselves to a deeper understanding of needs that are beyond survival, self-care, love, connection. We understand that life is not just about surviving on a practical level, we intrinsically know we need more in life. More fun, more connection, more time to ourselves, more reflection and all other things that bring us joy.

Being able to hold and touch another is the deepest intimacy we ever experience. To be able to stay present, in our hands, as we caress, is one of the deepest forms of bonding to another human there is. To feel the temperature and softness of another's skin, to place our hands in intimate areas, is to truly feel someone present next to you and to know your partner deeply.

BABKIN REFLEX

The Babkin Reflex makes the connection between hand and mouth. It works in conjunction with the Feet Hands and Face. Initially our hands want to bring everything to our face, including our feet! As mentioned, it plays a huge role in developing bonding and attachment, however it also plays a part in the development of fine motor skills of hand movement and manipulation.

When the Babkin Reflex is not fully integrated, we may see low proprioception in the hands, dropping things, clumsy hands and low tactile awareness. The mouth and face are also affected, and we can see facial tics and mouth movements, when fine motor skills are required in the hands, and dribbling/drooling. Eye contact may also be an issue specially as when in use, the eyes will need to be on the hands for effective use of them in complex tasks.

Emotionally, without the Hand Reflexes being fully integrated we will feel disconnected, clingy and insecure, being unable to trust and therefore form healthy bonds and relationships. It can lead to us feeling on the outside of the world and being defensive of who we are in ourselves, having to justify our behaviour to ourselves constantly. In more stressful times this can lead to compulsive habits, OCD and over thinking.

To check for the Babkin press lightly on both palms with your thumbs, then squeeze the forearms and squeeze the upper arms. While squeezing, notice what the fingers do. Do they curl in, and if so, how? Are the thumbs inside the other fingers or over the other fingers? Are they to the side of the other fingers?

TECHNIQUES TO INTEGRATE THE BABKIN

Weighted Hands

Place a weighted bean bag in the centre of the hand and close the fingers around it. Leave the weighted bean bag in the hands until you see the fingers visibly relax.

Hook-up Breathing

Cross arms and legs and place hands under your armpits. Breathe in and out with tongue on roof of mouth. On the next few out-breaths, relax your tongue. Repeat a few times. Next, uncross hands and legs and place fingertips together and breathe in and out in the same way.

Hand Stretches

Open your palms out as wide as you can, stretching the webbing between your fingers, then squeeze the hands together.

PALMAR GRASP REFLEX

The Palmar Reflex is more about grasping and clinging. It is thought to be a survival response to be able to cling to your mother, perhaps left over from our primal origins. This Reflex is much more important for healthy bonding, attachment and for communication through signing, speech, drawing, and writing. Without it, we find it difficult to translate what is in our heads out into the world, whichever skill we wish to use.

A retained Palmar Reflex will look like the tightly clenched fists we see in infants. Especially in times of stress, the hands will ache from being held so tightly. There may be constant tension in the hands, leading to painful muscles. This tension may extend up the arms to the shoulders, neck and facial nerves, especially the jaw joints. Tension in this area will affect the cranio-sacral rhythms of the body, inhibiting a deeper relaxation.

A retained Palmar Reflex will bring difficulty with handwriting and pencil grip, a tendency to drop things and poor hand dexterity. There will be challenges mastering fine motor skills like doing up buttons or shoelaces. In the mouth it will bring speech difficulties including stammers, jaw tension, teeth grinding and ultimately headaches.

Emotionally, we see feelings of anxiety and the consequent withdrawal and emotional disconnection. There may be a difficulty with empathy and awareness around other people's emotions as our emotional state is so all encompassing. Over long periods of time withdrawn and anxious, we can feel trapped and isolated, very lonely, even when we have a partner.

In more extreme cases, when this Reflex is retained, it can lead to increases in neurotic tendencies: phobias, OCD and self-absorption.

INTEGRATING THE PALMAR REFLEX

Paper Scrunching

With one hand, scrunch a piece of paper as small as you can and then open it out and smooth it flat again. Repeat with the other hand. Repeat as many times as you wish.

Palm and Finger Play

Palm side up, run a paintbrush from the centre of the palm in a spiral towards the outer edges. Then run the paintbrush along the inner knuckle from the small finger side to pointer finger side a few times. Next, run the paintbrush up the thumb pad, up the thumb to the tip. Repeat for each finger and on both hands.

Hand Outline

Starting at your wrist on your thumb side of the hand, pretend you are drawing an outline of your hand on a piece of paper. Move up towards the top of the thumb, down to the webbing between thumb and first finger, up to the top of the first finger and continue until your reach the wrist by the little finger.

Hand Massage

Using your thumb, press at the centre of your palm and work your way towards the edges of your palm. Repeat a couple of times. Then at the base of your hand, press a line up the palm and through to one of your fingers, giving a little extra pressure at the tip of the finger. Do this for all five fingers.

Case Study

One of the most satisfying clients that I have worked with, was also the most difficult. Steven is a boy who was born with many disabilities and has had multiple epileptic episodes, some major, some minor throughout his life. When I first met him, he was curled up in bed, unmoving, like a baby still in a womb even though he was 10 years old. There was little movement or connection to his body, and it was hard to know what kind of life he was experiencing.

Steven had done yoga with his mother in his early years, and his mother had even trained in a special method suitable for his depth of disability. But over the years, as no progress had been made, enthusiasm had worn off. Particularly, his mother told me, because she felt she was always 'forcing' him into positions, and he often grunted or complained in some way that indicated to her he was not enjoying 'being moved about.'

My first port of call, as is usually the case, was to work with the Feet, Hands and Face Reflexes. But it was with the hands that I first saw the results. Steven's hands were often in a tight fist, so much so that one of the ligaments on one of the hands were extended and his wrist was at all the wrong angles. There was no movement at all in the fingers or the arms.

After a few weeks of work, specifically on the Feet and Hand Reflexes, the mother began to report that his fingers were moving when he was having music therapy. A first! Over the coming months, his hands began to unclench, and I was able to massage more fully in the palms of his hands. Then, even more obviously, his arms started to move, and we had bigger movements in his eyes. Suddenly there were moments when it felt as if I was being watched, as I worked on his hands. And occasionally Steven would snatch his hand back when I was 'tickling' his hand with a paint brush. These signs of life were bringing Steven out of his inner world and into the wider world at last.

HAND REFLEXES AND YOGA PRACTICE

As with the Foot Reflexes, once integration has occurred at the beginning of your session through a massage or a hand stretch for example, it is now good to bring a little bit of extra attention to the hands. Perhaps feeling the air passing through the fingers as you move your hands in the air or 'drawing' an arc with your hands, so you are moving with complete awareness of where your hands are in space.

When doing weight-bearing exercises, one can begin to look more closely at where the weight is in the hand and how it feels up the arm. You can move your weight around the hands (like the funny feet exercise in the previous foot section), while you are in a yoga pose, and then ask what it feels like when you centre your weight in your hands again.

We need to remember that our first point of integration is raising awareness of what is happening in the hands, as we move and do our yoga poses. Once awareness has been heightened, we can remind ourselves to remember the pleasant feelings we had when integrating earlier in our session, so that the hands can relax and unclench or feel into the pose properly.

Please feel free to visit **www.the-empowered-feminine.co.uk** for a hand-based yoga practice example. At the end of this book, there are details as to how to access the videos that accompany this book.

Raising Hand Awareness: Finger Hugging

To begin, open and close your hands, perhaps giving them a stretch too, in time with your breathing. Breathing in, open the hands out wide. Breathing out, close them in again. Repeat a few times.

Now open a palm and place the thumb in the centre of it and close your fingers around the thumb. Take a breath. Be mindful of the warm 'hug' of the fingers around the thumb as you breathe. Open up the palm. Place your first finger and let the other fingers now hug this finger. Feel the warmth of your palm and the fingers on the first finger as you breathe in and out. Now keep going for all the other fingers of this hand.

Repeat for the other hand as well.

If you find awareness of your breath difficult, you could count to three for each finger or say affirmations, one for each finger, such as, "I am Safe, I am calm, I am happy, I am here, I am connected."

Once finished, sit with your palms open on your lap and keep your awareness on the centre of your palms for as long as you can.

AFFIRMATIONS:

"I am able to hold and keep what I need."

"I am opening to my experience of life."
"I have a choice to let go or hold on."

"I am who I am. I am free to be me."

"I can hug myself."

OTHER ACTIVITIES FOR INTEGRATING HAND REFLEXES

- Hand actions with nursery rhymes.
- Learning to Knit or Crochet.
- Learning an instrument that uses the hands and fingers (piano, wind, strings).
- Gymnastics (especially hand stands and cartwheels)'

THE MOUTH AND FACIAL REFLEXES

Our first connection to the outside world once outside of the womb is through our mouth. Our Facial Reflexes ensure we get our first nutrition from breast feeding and therefore survive without an umbilical cord. This transition from internal nutrition to external nutrition is the basis of Mouth Reflex work.

After the initial establishment of feeding routines and knowing we are surviving, the Mouth Reflexes become important parts in our exploration of the world, as soon everything is brought to the mouth and chewed, sucked and felt. When the need for oral stimulation is not met, the Mouth and Face Reflexes can become overactive, leading to constant movement in the face and mouth, oral seeking (like smoking for example) and can cause disruptions to learning and communication.

Facial expressions will be very responsive to internal and external stimulus and changes in the body and the environment, and all of this will be evident in the face. If heavily retained, the Facial Reflexes will result in symptoms like tics or Tourette's.

THE ROOTING REFLEX

The Rooting Reflex allows a baby to search for, find and open its mouth to then attach to its food source, the breast. Once the baby has this Reflex in place, the baby's Suck and Gag Reflex are activated, which also allows the baby to explore the world through its mouth as mentioned in the Babkin Reflex above. The Rooting Reflex is strongest immediately after birth and is seen as the baby turns its head from side to side looking for food. If the baby is not given the opportunity to root around for its food, this Reflex can stay stuck and cause problems with feeding, bonding and ultimately speech. The trigeminal nerve will become tense, and this can cause face/jaw/head pain, making biting and chewing and other motor functions sensitive.

With a retained Rooting Reflex, we may see thumb sucking and sensitivity to touch around the face and mouth. Oral seeking and chewing of objects like sleeves or a rag, teddy or toy. Later on, you may see speech difficulties and general discontented outlook to life, followed by poor self-esteem and even addictive behaviour.

INTEGRATING THE ROOTING REFLEX

Tongue Love

Pause for a moment and have a sense of where your tongue is placed in your mouth. Now place your tongue on the roof of your mouth (upper palate) and then move it to the lower palate and repeat a few times.

Now place your tongue on the inside of your cheek and move it from one cheek to the other cheek and repeat a few times.
Draw a figure of 8 on the inside of the gums with your tongue.
Draw a figure of 8 on the underside of your palate with your tongue.

Tongue Breathing

Cooling Breath. Roll the tongue into a tight roll in your mouth and breathe in and out through the tube it makes 3 times. Note that this isn't possible for everyone physiologically, so don't worry if your tongue can't do this.

Face Tapping

Using both hands, take your fingertips to the side of the bridge of your nose and tap out, following the cheekbone to the outside of your eyes. Continue tapping up to the temples, over the brows to the middle of your forehead and back out towards the temples, the corner of the eyes and towards the nose where you started.

THE VISUAL REFLEXES

The Facial Reflexes are very connected to the Visual Reflexes and are being integrated at the same time. This very primitive

Reflex System enables us to focus on near and distant objects, controls the size of the pupil in the eye and the cornea lubrication system which protects the cornea (blinking).

If these Reflexes are not well integrated or are overactive, they can cause excessive blinking when there's a sudden bright light or the forehead is touched. Later in life, when under a lot of stress, the eyes become hyper-responsive, resulting in tired eye syndrome, headaches and visual tics. You may have difficulties maintaining eye contact, and when there is eye contact, the jaw is tensed. You may feel dizzy, nauseous and teeth grind. You may experience motion sickness and spatial awareness alongside low proprioception, leading to breath holding or hyperactivity when in new environments. This may cause a resistance to changing an environment you are comfortable with in the first place. In more extreme cases, you may be compulsive sensory seeking, which may lead to being overloaded with sensory information.

INTEGRATING THE FACIAL AND EYE REFLEXES

Head Turning

Lying on the floor, place a visual aid (a toy or a ball) either side of your head at eye level. Turn the head slowly and rhythmically from one side to another letting your eyes land on the visual aid each time.

Stroking

With light touch, stroke your brow line starting at the centre of the brow and out towards your temple. Start with one eye and rhythmically do alternate sides between 8-10 times.

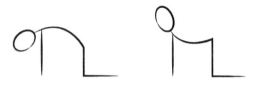

In all fours position with hands and knees on the floor, lift the head up and arch your back down as you breathe in. Look up to a point on the wall or ceiling in front of you. As you breathe out, tuck the head and tail in and arch your back up so you can look at a point either between your legs or on the wall behind you.

Raising Visual Awareness: Use your memory

Sit comfortably and find a visual picture to suit your mind and mood. It can be anything, however, a mandala works well for this exercise. Place the mandala a comfortable distance away from you and at a height that is comfortable for you to stare at. Let you gaze settle on the mandala and allow your attention to come fully into the present moment. Allow yourself to just be here taking in all the shapes, colours and form of the mandala, blinking when necessary, until you feel ready to close your eyes. When you have closed your eyes, begin to see if you can remember what the mandala looked like using your inner vision. Remind yourself of all its colours, shapes and form. Place the tongue onto the roof of your mouth and remember one of the integration exercises for vision above. See if this helps to keep you focused and present.

Case Studies

The story of Steven above continued with the Face Reflexes. At the same time as Steven's hands were coming back to life, there were changes in his Facial Reflexes as well.

When I first met Steven, he had a suction machine to collect all the saliva as he was unable to swallow and often dribbled and choked. Choking was very worrying as it was most distressing to watch. His clothes and pillow were often wet and uncomfortable and there was a lot of washing and changes of clothes involved in his daily care.

Within a few months of working with his Hand and Face Reflexes, I was told that the suction machine was hardly ever used anymore. I found that there were no more wet patches on his pillow or clothes, and more interestingly, he was developing a Swallow Reflex, so there was no choking at all.

He also ground his teeth less and beautifully surprisingly, he had a semblance of a smile coming in as the new, constant watching as I worked continued. It really was a joy to behold as I felt some bonding and connection developing.

MOUTH REFLEXES AND YOGA PRACTICE

Once the Mouth Reflex has been integrated using some of the exercises above at the start of your practice, we will find ourselves hyper aware of our jaw and our teeth and will notice whenever we tighten, swallow or clench our teeth during our yoga practice. We now know however, how to release this holding pattern and it can be very useful during yoga practice as we often will find ourselves holding here. Particularly if yoga poses are asking more from us than we find comfortable to do. Even then, in easy poses, as the mind begins to wander and become more active, most of us will find our mouth doing something. So, if we can continuously bring attention to what is going on in our mouth, we will find a myriad of ways to remind ourselves to release and then notice how this feels throughout the rest of our bodies, right down to our hands and feet.

It is a fantastic exercise to try to do a Sun Salutation for example and keep a constant attention on your mouth and jaw and watch how easily we slip into tension here. And if we are able to slow down enough, we will have time to remind ourselves how we have learnt to let that tension go through the work on Mouth Reflex Integration.

It is also a good practice to begin a yoga pose in an easy position – let's say standing forward bend – and then introduce a stronger stretch (working the hamstrings more). Then have another look at the jaw and mouth, only to find that we have clenched our teeth again!

One of the most effective techniques for observing the power of the Mouth Reflexes for me has been in Yoga Nidra. Once awareness and relaxation has been achieved in the rest of the body, coming back to the mouth and remembering the release pattern we had in the integration exercises will help most people quiet down their mind and find some relief from the chattering mind. Here more than anywhere else, the power of Reflex work is most obvious to most people.

You can use the meditation given above, in the Visual Integration section, titled 'Raising Visual Awareness: Use your memory,' as a Yoga Nidra practice to help integrate the Mouth Reflexes.

AFFIRMATION FOR FACIAL AND EYE REFLEXES

"I love what I see in myself."

"I see the world and all its colours, and I feel safe."

"What I see is a mirror in me."

"I see change and change is good."

OTHER EXERCISES FOR INTEGRATING YOUR MOUTH REFLEXES

- Learning to whistle.
- Blowing up balloons.
- Face Yoga.
- Consciously chewing your food.

IDEAS FOR YOGA PRACTICE USING FEET, HANDS AND FACE REFLEXES TOGETHER

So far, we have looked at these Reflexes in their individual capacities. However, we really want to bring awareness and attention to these all at the same time for the powerful effect these Reflexes integrated together can have. In this section, I will give ideas and examples of how to do this within a yoga class. These are of course, just examples of how you can use this work. As a teacher or practitioner, you may find that other ideas come to mind as you are practicing, and these can be just as powerful. You may find yourself using the integration techniques in other modalities as well, and they will be equally powerful. These examples all assume that integration work has happened at the beginning of the class in all three of these Reflexes.

METHOD 1

One way of using all three Reflexes simultaneously is by continually bringing your attention to either the hand, foot or mouth one at a time and then all at once.

Depending on the yoga pose, the pose itself will dictate which one to start with.

For example, in a pose like the bridge, the feet are beginning the movement (by being pushed into), so this is an obvious place to bring attention to. The hands can then be brought in, either by gently feeling the floor through the palms or by bringing the hands onto your back and feeling the material of your clothes. Then check in with your jaw, mouth and throat. Are you holding tension, is the jaw slack, what is happening in the mouth?

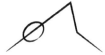

With a pose like Downward Dog, where hands and feet are already on the floor it is an easy thing to bring yourr attention to them. Most people are unable to touch their feet to the floor so having bean bags under your feet or a block to rest the feet on is helpful. However, bring your attention to hands and feet simultaneously, and your attention there as you check how your jaw is doing. Then once again, feel your feet and hands and face.

If it helps, work through in your mind's eye some of the Mouth Reflex Integration exercises whilst in the pose. Remind yourself of the exercises you did earlier on. Using the mirror neuron network works well with the Mouth Reflexes as often, our hands are not available to help as they are busy holding us up. Does anything shift anywhere? Do you feel it in your whole body? Other postures that can be used in this way are:

Baby Pose

Back Bend with Hands on Back

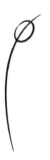

Warrior 1

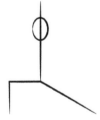

Shoulder Stand

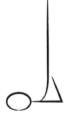

You can even split a session into three distinct sections. Integrating the Foot Reflex first, then doing some yoga around this. Moving towards integrating the Hand Reflexes, doing some yoga around this and then doing Mouth Reflexes. Towards the end of the class, you can then do a few poses where all three are being used at once as in the examples above.

METHOD TWO

Another way of bringing your attention to the FHF is to use the Hand, Foot and Mouth Reflexes as a way of bringing proprioception online. It helps us to understand where our body is in space and how the feet and hands and face are helping to bring this information to the frontline of our attention. Using the extremities like this, as a way of placing the body in space, is inherently relaxing and produces a mindful practice.

With every pose you try, tune into where your feet, hands and face are placed. If you are quite visual, you may see a drawing of yourself internally. If you are more kinesthetic, you may feel the feet hands and face as the ends of your body.

A yoga pose that this works very well with is Standing Forward Bend. With eyes closed, feeling your feet and hands, start to move your hands through space and bring them above your head so that they touch. Have a moment to think about the touch of feet to floor and hands to each other. Then as you fold forward, feel the weight shifting on the feet, the hands moving through the air and once in the final position of the fold, check in with the mouth and face. Is it relaxed? Is the jaw letting go? How does that affect the neck?

This principle is also very good for any sequence of yoga moves like the Sun Salutation, if done slowly and mindfully. Keep all the attention on the feet, hands and face, as you work through the sequence as appropriate.

Other poses that make this a good method to use are:

Swan Pose

Cobra to Downward Dog

Sitting Twists

Head Rolling

METHOD THREE

A third way of doing this, is to have feet and hands touching and continually bring attention to this touch, the heat, the sensation of palm to palm or foot to foot. Then, if possible, you can ask if both soles and palms can be felt touching simultaneously. Once this is established, bring in the awareness of the mouth and face.

A pose like Sitting Forward Bend has the added advantage that you can touch the ball of the foot to the palm of the hand. Having integrated the hands and feet and having your awareness heightened there, it is very comforting and relaxing to feel them touch each other. It can allow you to really begin to relax in the pose and have a more organised sense of what relaxing in a pose like a Forward Bend feels like.

Another pose where this works well is the Cobbler Pose. Having the feet sole to sole and bringing the hands to touch each other at the heart centre, or to touch the top of the feet feels amazing. Keep the awareness there as you breathe and relax.

Other poses that work with this method are:

Baby Pose

Chair Pose, with hands touching above the head.

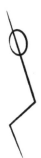

Squats with Hands in Prayer Pose

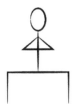

Turtle Pose

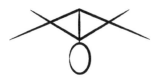

HAND FOOT MOUTH AWARENESS

Once you have done some movement as above, you can then explore this in a much more still environment. A good stillness practice that goes well with this is a simple body awareness, where your awareness is kept on the soles of the feet and the palms of the hands at the same time, for a period which feels right and depending on how much time you have.

You could make this more elaborate by beginning to draw around the outline of your feet and hands and exploring your face and mouth in more detail.

Start by bringing your attention to your right big toe. Find the very tip of your toe, and in your mind, start drawing a line down towards the foot and then up the second toe, around the top of the toe and down towards the foot and so drawing an outline around the third, fourth and little toe. Continue drawing your attention around the edge of your foot towards the heel, around the heel and up the instep towards the big toe. Join your attention to where you started at the big toe now being completely aware of the entire outline of your right foot.

Now do the same for your left foot. Bring your attention to your left big toe. Find the very tip of your toe and start drawing a line down towards the foot and then up the second toe, around the top of the toe and down towards the foot and so continue drawing an outline around the third, fourth and little toe. Continue your attention around the edge of your foot towards the heel, around the heel and up the instep towards the big toe. Join your attention to where you started at the big toe now being completely aware of the entire outline of your left foot.

Move your attention to the tip of your right thumb. Feel your attention move down towards the inside of your thumb.

Once you are in the flow of having the feet and hands and mouth in your awareness, you will find that you can be quite creative as to how you bring this awareness into your practice. All the yoga poses in one way or the other will have an element of this Reflex which makes it one of the easier ones to teach and bring into your practice.

Please feel free to visit **www.the-empowered-feminine.co.uk** for a hand-based yoga practice example. At the end of this book there are details of how to access the videos that accompany this book.

CONCLUSION

The feeling of safety and bonding within the body, feeling secure in one's skin and not feeling perpetually in danger will have an enormous effect on one's life. As this is a direct body-mind-spirit experience, it is difficult to describe, and it will be unique to you and your experience. Yet the feeling will be a positive one, bringing joy. There's nothing like embodying, "Everything will be OK. I belong, I am me and I am good," for your perspective of the world to change completely. Imagine being able to carry this feeling so deep inside your operating system, that it is so normal you don't even know it is there, and that it is a constant in your life.

For those of us who have suffered trauma or are on healing journeys of another kind, this foundation in ourselves, in our nervous system, can be the one thing that keeps us on track, even when it is hard, and we are having to look at difficult aspects of our psyche. The inner knowing that we have, that we are on the right track, that we are held and loved and guided, comes from this ability to belong, love and bond with ourselves. As we cultivate our body to feel this viscerally, so the mind will begin to acknowledge the truth inside of us. We are loved. We are safe. We are one with all.

WILD GEESE

You do not have to be good.
You do not have to walk on your knees
For a hundred miles through the desert, repenting.
You only have to let the soft animal of your body
Love what it loves.
Tell me about despair, yours, and I will tell you mine.
Meanwhile the world goes on.
Meanwhile the sun and the clear pebbles of the rain
Are moving across the landscapes,
Over the prairies and the deep trees,
The mountains and the rivers.
Meanwhile the wild geese, high in the clean blue air,
Are heading home again.
Whoever you are, no matter how lonely,
The world offers itself to your imagination,
Calls to you like the wild geese, harsh and exciting —
Over and over, announcing your place
In the family of things.

Mary Olive

CHAPTER 3

Fear Paralysis Reflex

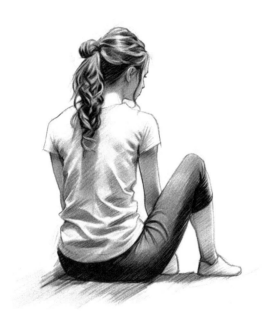

This Reflex is the first Reflex that most people initially can properly feel the impact of in their bodies. The Fear Paralysis Reflex (FPR) is one of the Survival Reflexes that we use the most in our yoga practice as it helps to move us from Sympathetic (Fight, Flight, Freeze or Fawn response) into Parasympathetic Nervous System mode (Rest, Digest or Relax response). One of our main outcomes in yoga is to help us reach a state of mindfulness and relaxation, both of which require the Parasympathetic Nervous System to be online. We are aiming to calm our stress responses, and this is what the FPR does beautifully. There is a big body of work out there on polyvagal theory and methods to activate this in the body. What most people don't realise is that the vagus nerve firing up is also determined by the Primitive Reflex System and it can be an automatic response.

This switch from one nervous system function to another is autonomic (automatic) and managed by the brain stem area of our brain. It is not always a guarantee that a yoga class will lead to relaxation for some people. In fact, for some, an intense asana led class can lead to over stimulation and an alert state. Those 2 minutes of lying down at the end can be torture for these people and the chances of really relaxing for 15 minutes or more are remote.

In these cases, the vagus nerve has not come online as it should because the yoga session was too intense and alerting, and the nervous system did not feel safe (Feet Hands Face Reflex) and consequently was unable to 'let go' into a relaxed state. Letting go into this state is difficult for many and as this switch is autonomic, we do need to remember that those with sensitive systems or PTSD may feel a loss of control, triggering them. This can lead to an even more alerted state or even a meltdown or PTSD episode so we must understand very well how to keep the system stable and safe (see Feet Hands and Face Reflex) and what to do if we find someone needing our help.

A great part of our training is dedicated to learning how to manage these reactions and so we do not recommend that you work with others. Experience it yourself and do more training if you are keen to share.

Once we have this knowledge, we can harness our training in the Reflexes to help everyone achieve the relaxed state that we are aiming for in our classes, especially those who have had difficulties and are unable to easily achieve a relaxed, open state.

When I have come across this Reflex in my students, my first impression is always of tension. I can see the tension in their bodies. There is a general overall feeling of the body being held in a trap, with a sense of it about to spring out, were it to be released. Like a wild animal with its whole body in a huge trap. However, the person themselves does not know they are trapped, this is normal function for them, and so they carry on, grumbling and complaining often about how their body aches. The tension is especially obvious in the curvature of the spine. It inevitably is in a C shape and seems to function as one solid unit. I also see the tension in the neck and jaw this causes.

Emotionally, there seems to be an unwillingness to share the inner emotions; it is better they are buried deep down where they cannot be experienced again. I have had a close relationship with someone whose way of processing emotions was to think about them deeply and meditate, perhaps, but not share much. Sharing caused the emotions to rise again and that was intolerable. If I ever asked how they were feeling, I was told. 'it was dealt with'. On the other hand, I was often told, "I wasn't understanding them," if they tried to explain what was going on. Connection was a real issue here.

I remember as a child, watching a close family friend of ours, go out into his garden and into his shed after a heated discussion with my parents. I always wondered what he was up to and on another visit had a peek into the shed when no-one was looking. Inside was a heater and a comfy chair, a safe little cocoon where emotions could be processed.

On the spiritual front, your ability to transcend the fear that is holding you back, is your ability to break free into a life outside of the metaphorical cave. You can begin to leave your ego-fear-thoughts behind and step into the light. An understanding of being held in the light and the Universe having your back, can descend and give you the confidence to move out of the rut you may find yourself in. You may begin to look for the people or modalities that finally help you break free. And even though your emotions may resurface to be dealt with properly at last, you know now that this is healing, that you need to go through this process in order to let go of whatever happened to you. In letting go, we begin to find ourselves in the present, able to make a new, brighter future for ourselves.

When I was first working on this Reflex for myself, I remember my first response was one of disbelief. I had spent, at this point, 10 years teaching yoga and I considered myself quite a relaxed person. What I hadn't realised was that I was using yoga as a regulation tool to keep me within the range of not going off the rails stress wise! Doing the integration exercises taught me to 'be relaxed' all the time. I was able to walk through life with a background feeling of 'everything is good, everything is always working out for me,' even if it wasn't, practically. When stressful moments arrived, I could take a breath, remember what the pattern in my body of relaxation was and, on the outbreath, recreate it in me so that I could move forward in that situation more present and less 'blown up'.

As time went on and the pattern of relaxation stayed in my body for longer and longer periods of time, eventually becoming the norm, being stressed again was out of the question. As soon as I felt the now not so familiar feelings of stress arrive, I would make a point of doing some integration exercises and finding the time for an intentional relaxation, Yoga Nidra.

The FPR is a Survival Reflex and is the first Reflex to emerge *in utero*. It forms the basis and neural patterning of our physical and emotional survival mechanisms. It is the base of the building blocks of our Primitive Reflex System, the first foundation to be laid. Therefore, it is the very base of our Central Nervous System (CNS). It connects the neural tubes and the beginnings of the spinal cord and is the very first response system to come online.

Before this, the embryo is many growing cells that have not yet responded to any stimuli from its environment. It is the most important Reflex to integrate and is very intelligent in how it forms the basis of our developmental system.

If the mother experiences stress or trauma in the early stages of pregnancy, this will influence the embryo. The embryo will respond to the stress alert signals on a cellular level and store these responses, creating a blueprint in the body/mind/spirit. This has subtle, lifelong effects on development, emotional and behavioural reactions and how we experience the world as human beings. The effect will be on the entire Primitive Reflex System, how it emerges and how the brain stem develops.

The next Reflex in line, the Moro Reflex, will also be affected as the FPR and Moro integrate at the same time. They are the basis of brain and emotional nervous system responses. The FPR connects the whole of the nervous system and stimulates the whole system to grow and develop. The very first discernible movements we make are made through the FPR activation and the foundation of our whole developmental growth is based on **movement**.

When the FPR is activated, it shuts down our entire system to help us survive the danger or threat (Freeze Response), whereas the Moro excites the system (Fight/flee Response). As the Moro helps the FPR to integrate, if neither are integrated, it can lead to low stress tolerance and hypersensitivity. There is a release of stress hormones, cortisol and adrenalin. In more extreme cases there is depression, excessive shyness, elective mutism and withdrawal from the world. Life is overwhelming and so to curl in and withdraw is the easier option.

When the FPR is in action, the body responds by curving in the spine and drawing in the legs, putting us in a 'foetal pose'. If not released properly in infanthood, the spine will have a pulled-in tailbone and will not be straight. The legs will be pulled in too, making these muscles in the legs and hips overworked. Sitting on the floor with the legs out in front of you or with crossed legs will be difficult and the spine will arch. There will be tension in the back, hamstrings, calves and Achilles heel. If this Reflex has been held since birth, telling someone to relax their back/hamstrings will not work. The muscles simply do not know how to let go.

The natural way to release the FPR Reflex is to be carried around and to be 'jiggled' as an infant. It always fascinates me how symbiotic the babies' developmental needs are with the instinctive responses of the mother. Picking up a baby and walking and jiggling them around to calm them is so intrinsic and it helps to release this Reflex. This is why baby carrying (in slings and backpacks) is to be encouraged over pushchairs and car seats. Especially in the first few months. The rhythmical movement of walking and jiggling the baby is the same as the rhythmical movement experience in the womb. Our mother's first walking movement is the very first thing our neural network perceives. It is how the network fires and connects. Therefore, active pregnancy is highly encouraged.

Children and adults with a retained FPR will have low tolerance to stress. There will be over-sensitivity to sensory input, and they will find it difficult to filter and process sensory information. All the senses will be delicate – from being picky eaters, to having motion sickness or visual disturbances. Under stress, there will be lack of eye contact, auditory information will feel overwhelming, including the sound of their own voice. The result of the sensory overload will be the beginning of a shutdown process, returning back to our first impulses of an immature stress response which is to freeze and withdraw. The stress hormones, cortisol and adrenaline, are released.

You can tell when the FPR is triggered as there is often problems with sleep and sleep routines or the opposite, not being able to be woken up calmly, as you may wake on high alert. There can be nightmares, night terrors and sleepwalking. Premature babies who have spent time in neonatal units will often have a retained FPR.

In adults, we may also see bad posture – low or tight muscle tone (especially in the hamstrings and back) and fatigue but especially, rigidity in the body. The body is sensitive to touch, sound and changes in the visual field, leading to disliking change and perhaps controlling behaviour to keep the environment under control.

The sensory system will instigate high anxiety, addictive tendencies and difficulties with being adaptable. We may withdraw from touch and develop compulsive, obsessive traits (OCD) and other phobias creating patterned behaviour we feel stuck in. Sometimes we are so stuck, we can't think or move at the same time.

Emotionally, we will have emotional blocks, low resilience and low tolerance with an underlying anxiety or negativity, leading to rigidity in our nature. As children, we will be clingy, and we will fear separating from a loved one. This will make our later relationships difficult, if we are able to have them, as we may be too insecure and shy, with low self-esteem, to even start them. Long term, this can lead to depression and isolation with fear of social embarrassment, social anxiety and fear of failure.

In more neurodiverse cases, we will see elective mutism, temper tantrums and hyperactivity with shallow, difficult breathing and breath-holding too.

The sad part is that children and adults with FPR want to be able to share their feelings and feel confident. They just automatically become frozen with fear and find it hard to thaw and share themselves. This is confusing, as we want to be one way but find ourselves unable to enact it, leading to more withdrawal from the world when we perceive we fail. Withdrawal is not always quiet. A child may scream loud and long, some to the point of going pale and exhausting themselves until they seem to pass out or sleep.

The vagus nerve is very much affected by the FPR. There is a lot of material available on vagus nerve toning, especially in the yoga spheres. So I will refrain from saying too much about it here. It suffices to say that it is the longest cranial nerve we have and that it runs all the way from the brain stem to part of the colon. It is then no surprise that all sorts of body processes are affected when this nerve is not toned up enough to do its job.

The main job of the vagus nerve is to connect the Parasympathetic Nervous System (our rest and digest mode). It slows our heart's beating and lowers our blood pressure; it controls how fast you breathe and even controls the muscle that contracts your bladder. When it's time for you to spring into action, it is the nerve that carries the signal to the brain to begin the process of starting the Sympathetic Nervous System mode, our mode of action. The information exchanges between the body and the vagus nerve affect the brain, the gut and your mood. Stimulating the vagus nerve has been shown to help with severe depression.

You can correlate here why it is that the FPR retention affects so many parts of the body-brain-spirit connection and we can also see how yoga, which gently stimulates the vagus nerve can be so helpful in FPR integration.

Try this gentle seated heart opening practice to feel the effects of the vagus nerve stimulation on you. Bring your hands to your shoulders. Inhale as you expand the front of your chest, open your elbows wide, and lift your chin. Feel your open heart.

Exhale as you contract your elbows in front of your heart and tuck in your chin.

Take several deep breaths like this. Focusing on your inhalation in this breath pattern can be uplifting. Allow yourself to expand into the open heart.

Please feel free to visit **www.the-empowered-feminine.co.uk** for a hand-based yoga practice example. At the end of this book there are details as to how to access the videos that accompany the book.

www.the-empowered-feminine.co.uk

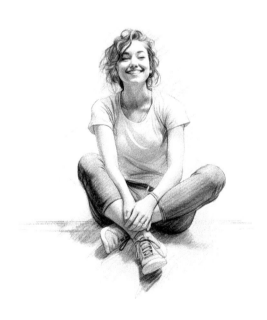

INTEGRATING THE FPR

At the beginning of this chapter, we saw how the FPR was originally integrated by the rhythmic movements in the womb and by being carried by our primary carer. Therefore, the movements that work to integrate the FPR are rhythmical and imitations of the natural movements we would have experienced in our early states of life. As we are that much larger and can no longer be carried, these movements have been adapted into a group of rhythmical rocking movements.

We also use powerful pre-birth movements which are slow and deliberate which re-enact movements from the womb environment. These moves in particular are very potent so I would recommend doing only one or two at the beginning of your FPR Integration journey.

RHYTHMIC ROCKING MOVEMENTS TO INTEGRATE THE FPR

Knee Bend Rock

Lying on your back, bend the knees and place your feet on the floor. Bring your awareness to your feet and direct the movement from there, gently pushing and pulling the floor away and towards you. Allow the body to become loose so that it is responding to this movement of the legs and feet, like a blob of jelly. Check your head can naturally move with the movement, including your chin bobbing along. Now begin to really focus on the rhythm you are moving at. Perhaps having a count, a song or a rhyme in your head you can move to.

Do this rhythmic movement for as long as you are comfortable but for a maximum of 2 minutes. When something changes, you may take a deeper breath, or feel a new sensation, or if you miss these queues, or feel a little woozy, stop and breathe and integrate. There will now be a new sensation coming in, sometimes quite strong in the beginning. Observe what is happening. This is the nervous system automatically switching into Rest and Digest mode. If it feels at all overwhelming, have a moment feeling your Feet Hands and Face. If you have worked on the FHF Reflex sufficiently, it will help stabilise the response. If you are unable to bring in the FHF, return to the previous chapter and spend another week integrating the FHF.

Ribcage Rocking

Place your hands one each side of your ribcage and gently rock yourself as if the ribcage were a big ball between your hands that you were gently patting side to side between your hands. Once you have managed to get some movement in the ribcage, concentrate on the rhythm you are developing and keep going until either your arms give in, you feel a change in the body or 2 minutes are up. When you stop, breathe and observe what is happening in your body. Use FHF if it feels too much to take in.

Knees-Up Rock

Lying on your back, bring your knees into your hands and lengthen your arms so that the elbows are straight. Let the hands hold your legs in place so that, were you to let go, the legs feel as if they could fall to the floor. Don't let go though! Now gently, using your fingers, start to rock your knees in your hands, pulling a little in and letting go over and over again. Let the body move to the rhythm you are creating in your hands and again find a song, rhyme or count you can continue to move to until you feel a change in the body, a new thought pattern comes in or anything else that may show your nervous system has had enough. As always, it's a 2-minute maximum. Again when you stop, breathe and observe your response using FHF if necessary.

PRE-BIRTH MOVEMENTS

With the Pre-Birth Movements, it is important to understand that although the rhythm is still there, it is now **extremely** slow. Imagine you are moving through treacle. The movements should be so slow they are slightly frustrating, but not so slow you are stop-starting, stop-starting. Try and develop a smoothness to the movement going as slow as you possibly can.

Cross Over Legs

Lie down and slowly, ever so slowly, lift one foot and cross it over the other at the ankle and then again very slowly place it back down resting the heel on the floor. Repeat this move a couple of times. Give yourself time to observe your response and use FHF if necessary.

Half Cobra Slides

Lie down on your back, and place the sole of your foot on your other ankle. Slowly, ever so slowly and deliberately slide one foot up the other leg bending at the knee as far as you can comfortably go and then slide it back down again as slow as you can. Repeat with the foot. Give yourself time to observe your response and use FHF if necessary.

Fist to Ears

Again, lying on your back place hands made into fists on your chest and slowly, ever so slowly bring them out and up towards your ears until you touch them and then slowly return them back to your chest. Give yourself time to observe your response and use FHF if necessary.

WHAT TO DO IF YOU FEEL YOU ARE FPR TRIGGERED

When you are highly stressed, in trauma or doing deep healing work, your FPR may get triggered. If there is a strong reaction to any of these movements, you may need some grounding first aid to help you calm your system down if the FHF has not been enough.

A hug or a squeeze works wonders, but if there is no-one around, a weighted bean bag or blanket will be just as good. You could do a relaxation (Yoga Nidra session, see videos) and use a bolster under your legs, lying your body on a cushion with your arms out to the sides in an open position. Or you could go to a wall and push against it, feeling your whole body working, paying attention to it, so you come back into your body fully. Place yourself in the room by feeling exactly where you are lying or sitting in comparison with the furniture, the walls, the windows etc.

OTHER EXERCISES FOR INTEGRATING THE FPR

Raising FPR Awareness: Butterfly Tapping

Sit quietly and cross the arms over the chest, bringing your hands together so that the tips of your thumbs are touching. Now start tapping slowly and rhythmically with the fingertips of one hand and then the other hand, onto the chest. As you work, let your awareness settle on your breath as you tap. Continue for a while, until you feel ready to stop. When you have come to a natural stillness, hold your hands over the heart and close both eyes with hands in a comforting position and settle into a peaceful state. Sit here comfortably and safely with the jaw and mouth relaxed.

AFFIRMATIONS:

"I am in the world."

"I am calm and present when I speak."

"I am well connected to my body and inner being."

"Nature is my friend."

OTHER EXERCISES FOR FPR INTEGRATION:

- Yoga Nidra
- Flotation Tanks
- Hanging upside down (yoga trapeze)
- Relaxation in a yoga trapeze or swing
- Floating in a Jacuzzi

CASE STUDIES:

There are multiple examples that I have seen work using this Reflex over the years, and many of them have been light bulb moments for the practitioners involved.

One of my favourites is from a long-term friend and yoga teacher herself, who had suffered years of chronic pain in her lower back. She told me, after a session at the Independent Yoga Network Conference, where I was teaching a class, that she had naturally found her own way of doing similar moves to alleviate her symptoms. She was pleased that she now had a more organised and purposeful approach she could follow which would help her even more.

FEAR PARALYSIS REFLEX IN YOGA PRACTICE

As most of the FPR moves are so relaxing, we need to give ourselves time to come up off the floor too, as the FPR rocking movements will feel heavy as the body is so relaxed.

Choose two or three integrating FPR moves to begin with and, having integrated the FPR at the beginning of your session, begin to bring it into movement and yoga asanas.

As this Reflex is all about relaxing the body, it is one of the easiest methods to use. The body needs to learn how to release the tension it has been holding and it is highly likely that there will be one area of the body that isn't able to release, even if it is something minor like an ankle that has been hurt in the past. If there has been any trauma to this area, or if this Reflex has been retained because of neurological differences, then there will definitely be tension to one or all of three areas.

The FPR targets three main areas of the body that hold tension: The hamstrings, the hips and the lower back. Some of the methods we can use to target these areas in our teaching and practice are given below:

METHOD 1

Hamstrings are a part of the body many people will find tight and uncomfortable. Often, they are tight even in people who are used to stretching them after exercise. If someone has a retained or unintegrated FPR, their hamstrings are bound to be tight and will often affect the sitting posture. Once an individual has learnt the FPR integration moves, their body will know how to relax the hamstrings. Using the mirror neuron network and our memory of what this type of relaxation feels like, we can begin to teach the hamstrings to release in a yoga asana.

For example, in a standing forward bend, the body will be struggling to fold from the lower back, the hamstrings will be very painful, and being able to relax will be quite hard. Therefore, you can take yourself in your mind back to the moment after your integration exercise where you first felt the body relax. Really go there and remember what that relaxation felt like and let your body feel that relaxation now (whilst you are in forward bend). Follow what happens in your body and keep observing what is happening and, 'like a wave,' follow it through your body.

This method is slightly easier when you are sitting down, so any sitting forward bends are good to start teaching this method.

Other yoga poses where this method works well could be:

Half Cobra Forward Bend

Push the Wall Forward Bend

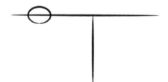

Warrior 1

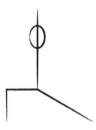

METHOD 2

Hip tension can lead to severe hip pain in older age, so working with the hips and learning to loosen them is very important. When there is hip tension, it can be in a specific part of the hip (front, back or side), or it can be in all parts. Therefore, a variety of hip related yoga practices are necessary to target all areas of the hips.

For example: Cobbler Pose

In Cobbler Pose, you can think about how to relax the legs down. Often this instruction is meaningless, so you need to have a practice first. You can lift your legs up and then drop them so that they 'bounce' or flutter like a butterfly... Lift your legs up and then let them go, as if they weigh a ton and they drop by themselves without your help. This may take a few tries. If it proves to be impossible, remember what it felt like after one of the integrations moves, you practiced at the start of the session. This normally works.

Once you have found some idea of relaxation, you can fold forward in this pose. This deepens the stretch, so you will need to concentrate even more on this 'feeling of release' practiced above. You can even visualise the legs being lifted and dropped again.

Another good example for this method is Alternate Leg Forward Bend (one leg straight, the other bent in Half Cobbler Pose). This gives you the opportunity to practice Method One and Two together as one leg can be doing Method One and the other Method Two.

Hips need to be stretched but they also need to be moved. Some of these poses therefore would need to be repeated multiple times. A good sequence for this is the Mermaid Sequence where the body is in constant movement. The mermaid sequence can be found in my Video series.

Other yoga poses where this method can be used are:

Hero Pose

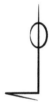

Side Stretch

 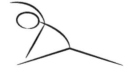

Cross Legged Twist

METHOD THREE

When working with the lower back it is important to be extra mindful. Lower backs are susceptible to being tight and getting tighter as you tend to pull in because of the pain. In fact, the lower back may tighten of its own accord just in anticipation of being stretched therefore starting with an idea of release is a good idea.

Stand and feel your legs relaxed into the floor. A little bit of Foot Reflex Integration or reminder is a good idea. Feel the support of the floor and to 'let the legs go into the ground.' The back will relax before you start, and this will be extremely helpful.

For example: Forward Bend

In Forward Bend/Fold you can feel your relaxed back as you start to move. And try to keep it relaxed as you move forward into the bend. When you feel your back tighten, stop, and in the position you have stopped at try and remember again how to relax the back. Then you can move forward again. When you are finally as far forward as you can get, once again remember your feet and how it felt to feel the support of the ground and to be able to relax your back.

METHOD FOUR

Because of the tension caused by the muscles around the lower back, the adrenal glands are often severely affected. Someone with FPR will be in constant flight or fight, so the relaxation of the adrenals is an important part of your yoga practice. Glands in general are released by a process of being squeezed and then stretched. As the endocrine system does not have a pump, glands are worked by being squeezed and released.

Bridge Pose and Wind Relieving Pose

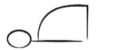

A good pose for this is going from Bridge Pose to Wind Relieving Pose a few times in a row. The squeeze in the Bridge is quite strong and so the stretch in Wind Relieving Pose feels a real relief.

A much gentler form of this method is Cat-Cow pose and any Back Bend to Forward Bend sequence works well. Cobra to Downward dog and back for example.

PRE-BIRTH REFLEX MOVES IN YOGA PRACTICE

When you integrate this at the beginning of a session, you will find that the session is extremely relaxed and probably would benefit from staying on the floor. Therefore, floor work, to begin with, is important.

METHOD 1 – FLOOR CONTACT

Feel the contact between your body and the floor and always move with this contact in the foremost of your mind.

Depending on the yoga pose you choose, this method requires that you move as slowly as possible coming in and out of the pose just as you did in the integration exercises and if the asanas flow from one into another then all the movement is slowed right down.

For example: Wind Relieving Pose

When moving into Wind Relieving Pose from the floor, feel the support of the floor, engage you core muscles and move as slowly as possible as you bring their legs towards your body. Breathe in the pose for a little while, long relaxing breaths, remembering how relaxed you were feeling in the integration process earlier. Then when it is time to move out of the pose, do the same: feel the floor, engage your core and slowly move your legs back down to the ground.

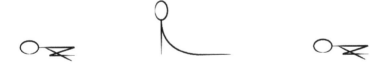

In a sequence like the Swan where you are going from Child Pose to Cobra Pose and back, you can move in as slow motion as you are able to. You can find the points where you have contact with the earth to help you keep the movement slow, but obviously, this can be quite hard work, so you will need to pace yourself as you see fit. As you come out of Child Pose, for example, you can feel the touch of the shins on the floor and the weight as it comes through the hands. As you either scoop forward or lie flat down (depending on your ability) the front of your legs will be in contact with the floor and the weight will come off the hands.

Remember that one of the aspects of Reflex Yoga that comes first into your consciousness is the heightened awareness of how your body is moving. And keeping that awareness between poses is as important as the pose itself.

Other poses that work well in a sequence are:

Any pose that does one side and then the other;

Floor Twist

Warrior 1 to Warrior 2

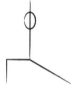 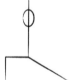

Side Stretches

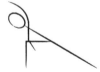

Any sequence of poses or poses that counterbalance one another.

METHOD 2 – OPPORTUNISM

Another method that the Pre-Birth Moves can be used in is what I call opportunism. Find a similar pose or one that does something similar to the Pre-Birth Moves and bring attention to it. This can be in either how the legs move, how the arms move or how the neck moves. Reminding yourself of this similarity and moving in the same way as when you were integrating the moves is very useful in any session.

For example: Tree Pose

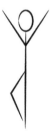

In the Tree Pose, instead of moving the leg straight up into position, rub your foot up your leg in a similar way as when they were lying down. Move just as slowly and really feel the touch of your foot upon the leg. Only bring the leg up as far as feels comfortable and stable. Now notice when the rest of the body wants to take part (the shoulders or jaw for example). If this starts to happen, then rest the leg right there and go no further.

Yogic Breath

When moving your arms in Yogic Breath, do this almost as slowly as when you were lying down doing a similar Pre-Birth Move. Breathe in as you bring your arms up, and out as you return them to your knees. Remember, the idea is to raise the awareness of the movement itself, and to keep it relaxed. So you could do this move as fits your strength and fitness levels, as well as to make the neuron connections. Here we are just taking advantage of the fact that some Pre-Birth Moves exist in yoga anyway.

CONCLUSION

Working with the FPR and the Pre-Birth Moves in yoga is one of the most satisfying of Reflexes to work with, as the results are visible in the practitioner straight away. If you look at the faces of those practising with you, you will see that they have 'sleepy' relaxed faces, and the eyes look like they have just got up from a deep sleep.

Many times, there are real 'wow' moments, as the body learns that it has been holding on to the legs or the back, as it releases for the first time in a yoga pose, for example. Once the system has relearned this release, it is rare that it will forget it again. Unless of course, there is an accident or trauma to this area again. Once recovery has happened however, the method can be reused, and the neurological pattern remembered again. The more times the body can use these integration exercises and learn this new patterning, the better it will be able to permanently stay in this relaxed state, not just in a yoga practice but in everyday activities too.

This is when you begin to see that the body is no longer returning to tension in the hamstrings, as the case study at the beginning of this chapter demonstrated. Now there can be progress, and week on week, a deeper loosening of all the holds that this Reflex has held onto for many years, and sometimes since birth.

In the emotional and spiritual states, the body will begin to feed the mind the information of being calmly in your body. This state of embodiment is a safe state to be in. Signals from your body will be of calm and connection. And you will be able to have the sense of being at home inside your body; and that this is a good place to be. The feelings in the body will be less stuck and more flowing. Perhaps even able to release pain and see it as an energy that is stuck, and now is beginning to move and flow. This can be reflected in life as well. Where before, aspects of living seemed stuck (like a dead-end job, for example), there will be change and a move forward in the direction desired. We begin to feel we can move towards change without fear and instead embrace it as an opportunity. These fear-based thoughts that used to hold you back, will now be acknowledged as just thoughts you don't need to give energy to. You may even begin to see that they aren't really your thoughts but were put there in childhood or by someone close. These thoughts don't belong to you and never did. You just adopted them. Now you can let them go. Now you can move through them to something new and grow into someone new.

SOUL MATES

I thought I would find you,

Come across you, see you some day.

I thought that through my eyes I would recognise who you were;

Now I understand that you are nowhere.

That when I close my own eyes,

Look within,

That is where I find you.

I always thought that when I kissed you,

Tasted you, absorbed you some day.

I thought the chemistry in me, would recognise the chemistry in you;

Now I understand you are nowhere.

It is here,

As I taste my own flesh,

That I find you.

I always thought that when you'd touch me,

And my body quivered,

Beneath your tender fingertips, I would know an angel was holding
me;

Now I understand that when I feel into my own body,

Acknowledge my own quiveryness,

That I find you,

In the end.

You are within me.

The moment I chose to be present,

Accepting and here in this moment, in the world around me –

That is where you reside.

There is the company I always sought;

You're here with me.

When they say 'love yourself,'

What they mean is –

Love this moment

And yourself in it.

Be here.

With gratitude in your eyes, a sweet taste in your mouth,

Centred in your body;

And understand that this is it.

This is life.

This is here and now.

This is, my friend;

This is where your soulmate lies.

Veronika Peña de la Jara

CHAPTER 4

The Moro Reflex

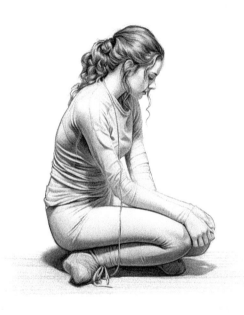

The Moro Reflex is a highly requested Reflex in Reflex Yoga, as it is the one that deals with high anxiety levels. Often, we are experiencing very high levels of anxiety, perhaps leading regular to panic attacks in day-to-day life, but think that there is nothing we can do about it. Once we realise this is something that can be alleviated, then the requests come flooding in. Our society has always berated those with mental health issues of any kind and often anxiety is a hidden problem, not talked about and not dealt with. We may feel that we are not ourselves, that we cannot function properly, and we don't know what is happening to us. Worry sets in that there is something deeply wrong with us and anxiety doubles and sets in for a long time to come.

It is often really comforting to know that what is happening to you is automatic and can be remedied. When you realise that this is part of your survival response, that you have no control over that response but that there is a way to calm that response down, suddenly you feel like you can help yourself and the feelings of helplessness go. This ability to have a tool in your toolkit that you can use to help yourself and others is empowering, and I have often seen how just knowing about the Reflexes has helped someone to regain enough confidence to move forward in their healing journey.

This Reflex is also very personal to me as I had this strongly, unbeknown to me, for many years. I believe it was triggered by a car accident I had as a 6-year-old. Although not a very severe accident, I was unlucky enough to be in the back seat between the two front seats. So when the car crashed into a suddenly stopping bus in front of us, I flew out of the car and hit the back of the bus with my head. I remember the feeling still, of flying through the air with my arms outstretched either side, taking a big breath in, and then all was black.

As a yoga teacher trainee, I always found Pranayama (breath technique) in yoga classes difficult to follow and would inevitably 'bluff' it. I looked like I was doing it but was getting agitated and I couldn't wait for it to stop. My earliest teaching never included breath cueing, or any Pranayama exercises. And I never even noticed that that was what I was doing. My body was unconsciously steering me away from controlling my breath in any way.

It is interesting that my first experience with panic attacks was with learning to dive. Underwater scuba diving brings with it breath awareness, as you can both hear the breath and feel it (as there is resistance due to the fact it is compressed air). In my initial training, whenever I had to take my diving mask off and cold water washed over my eyes, my breath would freeze, and I would panic and swim for the surface. It was a blind reaction and at the time I thought it was related to trauma from a near drowning when I was 3. When after the 10th time reaching for the surface, my instructor told me I would fail the course if I didn't hold it together, I finally controlled that reaction and forced myself to breathe calmly. This got me through my training, and I eventually became a dive guide (divemaster) and in the end, enjoyed messing about with my breath underwater. This was a really empowering moment in my 20-something self, and it taught me a lot about my own inner strength, even though I wasn't sure how I had managed it or why I had a problem in the first place! Not long after, I discovered yoga.

Working on the Moro Reflex has affected my body posture. What I thought was a family gene that made the women of our family curl inwards at the breastbone was a pull from a very tight diaphragm. As a yoga teacher I was always aware of this 'fight' to stay upright in my body. I clearly remember going to my first yoga festival as a young teacher and thinking I was in trouble now. In class I could be mindful to keep myself upright. However, here I was surrounded by yogis who were just chatting, eating, laughing, all in a perfectly naturally upright position, I could only master with full awareness! I didn't understand or know then that its uprightness wasn't something you had to do; it happens naturally when your diaphragm is relaxed! I also hadn't realised that when I was particularly upset or tense, I would also hunch my shoulders and as my friend would say 'look like a gorilla.' She could always tell by this stance that I was triggered by something.

My most enlightening discovery about the effect the Moro was having on me has been more recent. I had always been good at working on all three aspects of myself: Body, Mind, Spirit. I was a yoga teacher, so my bodywork helped raise awareness of my body, daily. I meditated so I was master of my mind. I could, with difficulty mostly, find a way to have a sense of something bigger than me, who I knew had been with me as a child. I could move between all these three states quite fluidly. What I hadn't realised was that these three states could co-exist within me simultaneously. Integrating this Reflex, really taught me that these three modes of being were one. I became whole once again after having been blown up into three parts most of my life.

It still took many years of practice to come to where I am now in healing my Breath-Trauma Response and the Moro Reflex. What I have learnt has not only done that but also helped me to progress all the other Reflexes above it that were stuck as a result.

The Moro Reflex is more commonly known as the Startle Reflex and is the one we most remember seeing in infants. Usually, they are asleep and there is sometimes a loud noise, and sometimes no reason at all, and the baby startles, throwing their arms back over their head, opening their hands and taking a big breath in and then moving the head forwards, closing their hands into fists and breathing out. This Reflex is designed for taking a breath in when the baby is born so that it can survive outside the womb. However, it is active inside the womb, as it helps exercise the breathing apparatus before it needs to be used.

Although its main function is for the breath, it also has a role connecting the upper and lower body together, connecting most of our brain structure, as well as the muscles used for neck and trunk control. Head control is important for overall development, as we will see in the following chapters. As a result of its role in head control, it also has input to the sensory system. It affects our sensory intake and processing and so is easily activated by sensory input such as unknown sounds, for example. How do we process a sound we do not recognise, especially if it's loud? If we can't, we will find ourselves on high alert.

The Moro can also be triggered by strong stimulation of the balance, auditory, visual or tactile/proprioceptive senses. The body is then in defence mode as the adrenalin, epinephrine and cortisol are secreted by the sympathetic nervous system. Epinephrine is particularly relevant here as it lasts longer than adrenalin in the body; and can keep it on alert for as long as 12 hours. This means that if there is even the slightest stress during those 12 hours (someone dropping a plate on the floor, for example), the body will begin a new 12-hour cycle of epinephrine. You can see then how hard it may be to calm the body down and how high stress can continue for days on end.

As mentioned in the last chapter, the Moro and the FPR work together to integrate each other. The FPR is more of an internal Reflex, alerting and responding to the internal sensory response world, whereas the Moro responds to the external, alerting world.

For a baby, this Reflex is their subconscious communication to reach out to their caregiver and to be somehow soothed when they find themselves alerted to 'danger'. If this nurture doesn't happen then we will feel unsafe, abandoned and isolated. The Moro therefore has an important role in our personal evolution and if unintegrated as an infant will be influencing us as children and adults. It can cause sensory disruption where one or more of the senses becomes highly sensitive and a need to 'flee' from external sensory stimuli is needed. Fleeing can take the form of hiding under the bed to disassociated states. Another response is to seek stimulation to flood out what is overstimulating, like listening to music on headphones or watching endless episodes of TV. For some there will be oscillation between these two states.

If we experience chronic stress or a traumatic incident, the Moro as an automatic response will become over-alert and leave us in a constant state of Fight, Flight, Fright response. The breath will be constrained at times of tension, perhaps leading to panic attacks and even misdiagnosed asthma. You will struggle with sport, for example, as the stress on the body will trigger the breath cycle into stress and your breath will give up before your body does. The tension in the breathing apparatus can lead to tightness of the muscles of the ribs, upper back, chest and shoulders which will contribute towards chronic fatigue syndrome and burnout in adults.

In children, we will see them unable to handle external sensory impressions and will withdraw into themselves to shut off the stimuli. They will become afraid to explore unfamiliar situations and will have outbursts of anxiety if there is a change or routine. There is a lack of inner security, so they are rarely spontaneous and may feel a need to dominate and manipulate playmates. If a child doesn't withdraw, then they will be over-excited (hyper) and constantly bouncing off their environment.

Adults may present themselves with a higher need for constant stimulation which could lead to addictive behaviour. They may need to have a lot of control over their situations and relationships. Or they may seek a lot of approval, be a people pleaser and have difficulties being alone, which could lead to being in vulnerable situations or relationships repeatedly.

The physical signs of a retained Moro Reflex are more than you would imagine. Apart from the one's mentioned with difficulties in breathing and tightness in the upper torso; frozen shoulder, low muscle tone in the upper body, leading to poor neck, head and trunk control, as well as back aches and over-extensions in the lower back, chest, arms and hands are common. The sensory system will have sensitivity and you may see this in dilated pupils, and headaches. There could be jaw tension, skin reactions and bowel problems like IBS.

The Moro Reflex is often more active when waking. You may even startle awake and feel emotional or angry for no remembered reason. This may lead to defensive, emotionally reactive behaviours and a rabbit in the headlights look – Moro people are not good morning people! The upper body may also feel tight in the mornings with difficulties in raising arms, clenched fists and moving the upper body as one unit, unable to isolate body parts. There may be pain in the tight neck and shoulders, difficulties with breathing and breath holding. In the evenings, you may appear to have dilated pupils and poor twilight vision.

Typically, in the emotional realm, we will see hypersensitivity, difficulties with change and unexpected situations which could lead to controlling, manipulative behaviour. More rarely, there will be a low will force, low self-esteem and feelings of abandonment. Add to that, difficulties in letting go, coping with criticism and connection to peers and we see emotional and muscle armouring in relationships.

In a learning environment, there may be poor attention spans, challenges with listening skills and language. And inside our own lives we may have difficulties with self-care, lack of impulse control and poor adaptability.

On a spiritual level, the Moro keeps us disconnected from self. We can become disassociated, loosing hours of our day to nothing important in an attempt to 'zone out' from the overwhelm we feel. We live life in a dream, hardly present, with a lot of brain fog. When we are in survival mode, it is much harder for the parts of the brain that allow us access to our higher states of connection to be online. We cannot focus or meditate. It is as if we were unplugged from the spiritual part of ourselves, rarely coming into connection with our inner being and our sense of 'oneness to all' We may put a lot of effort into trying to make these connections only to find ourselves asleep or distracted.

The Moro Reflex is closely connected to the development of the Limbic System in our brain. The Limbic System processes and regulates our emotional biochemistry and memory. It influences our mood, motivation, our pleasure and pain sensations, and our ability to feel stable and socially connected. From the very beginning, the Moro is the connection between nature-nurture, our ability to seek protection from our mother and instinctually ask for what we need. It greatly affects our emotional development and response throughout our lives.

The Limbic System receives information from our inner environment and our outer surrounding world in the form of emotions. Our inner organs, our vagus nerve and our sensory perception all influence our thoughts and emotions. One of our most important developmental journeys is to develop the ability to self-regulate and be able to understand our own needs and act accordingly in a balanced way. Perhaps calm us down, feed us when we are hungry or cheer ourselves up. If the Moro has stayed active, the Limbic System cannot perform this self-regulating role effectively.

An overactive Moro will also result in low feelings of the heart, low empathy, compassion and low gratitude. For this reason, keeping the heart area warmth and having a daily gratitude or compassionate practice can be very helpful. There are many practices of this kind readily available for you to try, my favourite is Metta meditation from the Vipassana tradition.

PERSONAL PRACTICE

Please feel free to visit **www.the-empowered-feminine.co.uk** for a hand-based yoga practice example. At the end of this book there are details of to how to access the videos that accompany this book.

www.the-empowered-feminine.co.uk

Begin by checking in with your body and your breath, and afterwards have a moment to tune into how different you feel – perhaps answering some of these questions:

1. How am I breathing? Where is my breath now compared to where it was at the beginning? Am I breathing deeper or more into my belly?

2. How is my body feeling? Where in my body can I feel the results of the work I have done? How would I describe this feeling and where it is?

3. How am I feeling emotionally? Has this changed from the beginning of the yoga session? How would I describe what I am feeling to someone else?

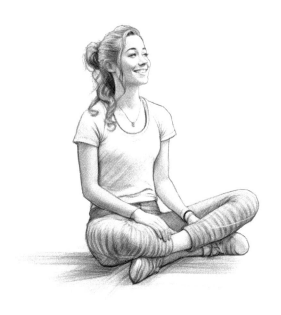

INTEGRATING THE MORO REFLEX

An infant will release the Moro Reflex through the nurture of their caregiver. Keeping the baby close to the mother's heartbeat, keeping baby warm and close and even placing a hand on the baby's chest will be helping to integrate the Reflex. There are rhythmical movements as babies are often kept close, carried on the chest or back, as the mother walks. However, there are other exercises which can help too, such as isometric pressure and certain copycat movements, of breath and coordination to help create heat in the upper body.

Spleen Rock

Wrap your arms across your body, right hand under the left rib, left hand on the right elbow, as in a hug. Gently start to rock your ribcage side to side. Use small movements and get into a rhythm, perhaps using a song, a rhyme or a count.

Keep rocking the ribcage – try to make it as easy and fluid as possible. Use only your hands and arms to move the ribcage, keeping the shoulders as relaxed as possible.

Keep going until you feel a change in your nervous system. It may be subtle, coming in as a sigh or a slightly deeper breath or it could be more obvious with a sudden rise in heat, flush of the face, or if a bit more extreme, a slight feeling of nausea.

If this occurs, remember to use FHF to stabilise your nervous system. Keep your arms wrapped around you to keep the diaphragm warm.

Isometric Moro Breathing

Lie down and place your hand on your solar plexus area. Take a deep breath in and feel where your diaphragm pushes your hand away. Now you know where your diaphragm is, next time you breathe in, hold the breath and gently push back with the heel of your hand – for a count of 3 or more, depending on your comfort. Then release the pressure with an exhalation. Again, repeat these two or three times depending on how it feels. Afterwards keep the hands and arms wrapped around you to keep the diaphragm warm.

Shoulder Rolling

Place your hands in front of you and imagine you have a bundle of clothes in your hands you are going to wash. Roll your hands with shoulders going round and round one way and then the other way. This looks very much like a salsa shoulder move. If you have difficulty getting this started, you can break it up into sections:

1. Imagine you have a bell just above each shoulder, alternately, try and ding each bell with each shoulder.

2. Imagine the bells have moved so they are now in front of your shoulders, alternately try and ding each bell with each shoulder.

3. Now try and ring all four bells, each shoulder going around in a circle, one side and then the other.

4. Over time you will speed up the circular movements until you can do both shoulders simultaneously.

WHAT TO DO IF YOU FEEL YOU ARE MORO TRIGGERED

Integrating the Moro Reflex can be very comforting for the individual, but sometimes you may find that you have become emotional and over done it. Whenever this happens, stop what you are doing and come back to the Feet, Hands and Face Reflex we covered in Chapter 2 and calm the system down. When this happens, most times it is better to stop all Moro work immediately and work on the FHF for a few more weeks.

If your system has become overloaded, you may experience red ears; you may do a series of yawns or notice an obvious change to your breath. If you over do it too much, you may become emotional or fidgety, have sweaty palms or an urgent need go to the toilet.

If you need more First Aid input, try getting a hot water bottle and keeping the chest warm. Lie down and feel the weight of the water bottle on your chest. You can also try humming a low hum for a few minutes or reducing sensory stimuli for a few moments; support your head, close your eyes in a quiet room.

OTHER EXERCISES FOR INTEGRATING THE MORO

Moro Relaxation

Lie comfortably on your back on something warm such as a sheepskin or rug and making sure your chest is covered and cosy. Raise your feet and rest them on a chair or sofa. Start to notice your breathing and keep track of it, without changing it, for a few breaths. Notice how your breath may be slowly deepening. Don't do anything to change it, just observe. Don't worry if you start to feel sleepy or lose track of your breath. Whenever you notice you have been distracted, return to observing your breath. Keep going for as long as you feel you need to.

AFFIRMATIONS:

"I am calm."

"I am safe and calm in my surroundings."

"I accept and enjoy everything as it is."

"I breathe in fresh air."

OTHER ACTIVITIES FOR MORO INTEGRATION

• Hot water bottles

• Saunas

• Breaststroke in swimming

• Once better integrated: Breathwork

Raising Moro Awareness: Hand Rubbing

Sit comfortably, making sure your whole body is warm. Gently rub your hands together, including rubbing between your fingers, until your hands feel warm and awake. Gently close your eyes and bring your awareness to your hands.

Begin on your right hand and feel the fingertip or your right thumb, first finger, middle finger, ring finger and little finger. Let your attention wander up all your fingers one by one through all the fingers to your palms.

Notice the warm palm of the right hand and the back of the hand and bring your awareness to the wrist. Feel the whole of the right hand from the fingertips to the wrists, all at once. Repeat on the left hand.

Once both hands have been in your awareness, try to feel both hands together, perhaps feeling both tips of the thumb, first finger, middle finger, ring finger and little finger. Feel all then fingers, both palms and back of the hands and both wrists.

Finish by feeling all of the right and left hands together.

CASE STUDY

As is often the case, when you have your own Reflex to integrate, you find yourself working with lots of others who are in the same position as you! I have had many clients on a one-to-one basis where the Moro Reflex has been the main issue they are dealing with.

My first ever case was with R who was in the middle of getting a divorce from a very dysfunctional and abusive relationship. The first thing she said to me as I worked out how to help her was that she felt she was on the edge of losing herself and that she was afraid she'd never find who she was before her relationship turned bad.

I remember this case so well because it was an immediate turn around. By the end of our very first session, when she came out of relaxation, she looked at me and I could see in her eyes that she was back. Without knowing her well, I could see the true relaxation that had come to her, and she said: "What you do is nothing short of a miracle. I never thought in an hour and half, I could be back to normal after years of suffering." We continued to work together until her divorce was through and her new life had happily begun again.

A more recent case is even more interesting, as I was working with H, who is recently diagnosed as ASD (Autism Spectrum Disorder), as women often are, very late in life. It was a beautiful day after our very relaxed and passive Reflex Yoga session and she asked if she could leave the car in my drive and go for a walk after our session (I live in a particularly beautiful AONB – Area of Outstanding Natural Beauty). She drives from quite far away, so of course, I had no issue with this.

She was gone for hours – to the point that I was slightly worried, as it was beginning to get dark! Anyway, when she did arrive back, I happened to be outside hanging wet clothes on the line. "It was blissful up there," she said. "I didn't want to leave."

The next day, I received a text asking the question: Could a Moro Reflex deprive one of bliss? Is that why I have felt moody and cantankerous all my life? I have never been as happy as I was on that hill yesterday. My whole body felt different, and I was HAPPY. Thank you.

The first time one experiences a new way of being from Reflex Yoga is always momentous. It's a glimpse of how life can be, and you never forget it. Then you get to work with the body, and you work towards something you now know exists!

THE MORO REFLEX IN YOGA PRACTICE

Many of the integration practices are intended to heat up the upper body and back, and this then affects the upper back, shoulders and neck. There are many methods that we teach in our Yoga Teacher Training, which help us warm and stretch the upper body. However, when working with the Moro, we also have to bring in the breath. Breathing can also have been compromised before integration and so you are left feeling a new freedom of breath. When working with yoga and the Moro Reflex there are two areas to consider. There are many methods that we teach in our Yoga Teacher Training which help us to marry the two practices together. Here are a couple for you to get an idea of how it works...

METHOD 1 – ACCENTUATING THE BREATH IN YOGA POSES

When using this method, it is good to have gone through the exercise of measuring breath volume before and after the integration exercises.

Close your eyes and breathe out completely.

Then taking a natural breath in, count gently as you fill up. Notice what number you are at when your lungs feel completely full. Also notice how it feels when you are full. Is it like reaching a brick wall? Is it tight in your chest?

Once you have a number in your head you will repeat this exercise after some Moro Integration to see the difference.

This way you will feel that you have made a difference in the way that you breathe, and you will feel your breath has expanded in some way already. Then you can use poses that help stretch the breathing apparatus. Try to breathe in an expansive way despite the stretching you can feel in each pose.

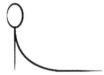

For example: Cobra Pose

Starting with the body face down, take a deep breath before you even start to move. See if you can feel any constraints already in your breathing as there is now weight-bearing on the diaphragm and chest.

Bring your hands beneath the shoulders and still without lifting the head, push the floor and feel the shoulder blades activate. Note if there is a difference in how you breathe now that there are muscles active.

Lift up your head to look up at the ceiling and breathe in. See if you feel any constraints in your breathing. Come down and rest.

Next before you come up for another try, remember one of the integration exercises and how it felt to breathe freely afterwards. Keep this memory as you come up into Cobra Pose again.

Repeat a few times so that you have a chance to feel this difference.

Other poses where this method works well are all chest stretching poses such as:

Yogic Breath

Warrior 2

Bow Pose

Bridge Pose

Fish Pose

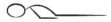

METHOD 2 – HEAT AWARENESS

The second method that is good to use, is to take advantage of the heat that is felt when this Reflex is released. When you do the integration exercises, draw attention to the heat that is felt deep inside the chest cavity. Work out which of the integration exercises has the best result and produces the most heat. Then when you are in a pose, use the heat you can feel to draw your attention to the area that needs help to be released.

For example: Seated Twist

Sit comfortably and relax your legs in a cross-legged position. Then step one foot over the other leg and bring the opposite elbow over the opposite knee.

Remind yourself to once again relax your legs, as you begin to twist around, feeling the lower spine turn first and then as you reach the upper spine, the Moro area, stop twisting and breathe.

Feel the heat that you remember you generated in the integration exercises. You could even image for a moment that you are doing the exercise again in your head, mirroring the previous integration work, whilst in the pose.

Then once the area is feeling the warm, see if you can move through the twist a little more.

Repeat on the other side.

This method also works with back bends in a similar way to Method 1. As you come into a cobra, for example, feel the heat generated from the integration exercises as you breathe into the pose.

Method 2 would also work with the following poses:

Floor Twist

Warrior 3 and 4

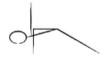

Bridge Pose

Fish Pose

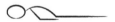

Cat-Cow Pose

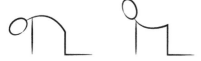

Side Stretches

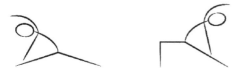

CONCLUSION

Integrating this Reflex has a profound effect on how your body feels in real-time. It is not until you have first experience 'the other way of being,' without this Reflex being active, that you notice how much stress and uncomfortable feelings you have been living with. I had someone ask me once after a session, "Can life really be this blissful?" For some, the first time this new pattern comes into their lives is also the first time they see a ray of hope that life is worth living. It is powerful to witness.

Now the body can keep calm, even when life around you becomes stressful. An extraordinary awareness of what is happening to the body and the breath arises, which you can then harness to help you, rather than it running away with itself into feelings of stress and being out of control. Here we can take a deep breath, take a moment and respond calmly to what is going on around us.

We are also triggered less easily and so can move through life with ease, without fear of being triggered. Our responses will be more measured, and we will be able to think through sequentially and in a centred way, how to respond. We will also make better decisions which have been considered, rather than ones 'in the moment,' which are just reactive. We begin to feel more able to control our words, and to use appropriate and less igniting words. We can keep our awareness fully in our body, even when conversations become hard, we can discuss and argue our point without getting upset.

Once we are more settled in our body, without fear of being destabilised, we are able to have more compassion to others. As we are not so reactive, we can perhaps see that other people's behaviour has nothing to do with us, and so we can open our hearts to their suffering. Compassion can flow easily. This includes having compassion for ourselves.

With a less reactive body, we can see that we are human and that sometimes we aren't capable of doing the right thing in a particular moment. However ,we can face up to our difficulties, apologise, learn and move forward with gratitude for our newfound capabilities.

This Reflex really helps us understand ourselves on the emotional level. We can see our patterns, what triggers us, how we respond and learn new, better ways of reacting. We finally have the space to sit back and ponder what the best course of action is, rather than running full tilt into a dramatic response. This means we make less mistakes when dealing with life, have better, calmer outcomes to our actions. We mature immeasurably and become more emotionally intelligent as a result.

KIND FACES

This host of kind faces
Smiles in unison as the knowledge sinks deep;
There is a wind of knowledgeable change
That Creeps in unseen.

Through all the storms and long summer days,
Through the cold winter dusk, sun setting,
Inside a fire-lit room:

Bodies have moved and removed.
Patterns have broken
And been remade new.
Laughter has echoed;
Heads have emptied
And the wind of knowledge
Has crept in unseen.

In-between the check-ins and the cracks of snacks,
Inside the notes, the highlighters track
Across the paper wide:

Minds have been shaken and rearranged,
Patterns broken
And thoughts made new.
Headaches have come,

Heads have gone,
And the winds of knowledge
Crept silently in.

Amongst the holding of hands and the sharing of hearts,
Between the love showers, the tears of support
Inside these human hearts:

Openings have come and trust renewed,
Patterns broken
And Love made new.
Friendships have blossomed,
Differences accepted,
And the life-force energy
Has finally crept in.

This host of familiar faces
Rises in unison as empowerment sinks deep.
There is a wind of knowledgeable change
that Creeps in unseen.

Veronika Peña de la Jara

CHAPTER 5

Spinal Galant

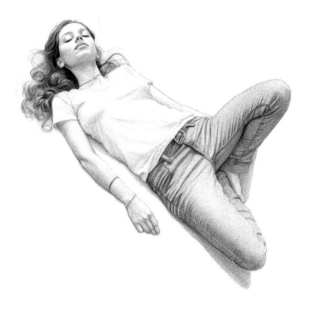

This Reflex is an interesting one in yoga as you will find that the few people who have it, who would benefit from doing yoga, rarely feel like coming to a yoga class! Sometimes they come with a friend and suffer through the session, wondering what others see in so much stillness and mindfulness, as it drives them potty. Perhaps they will even have a giggle and will shake themselves off, like a dog, during the class, trying to land in their bodies in their own way. Instead, we tend to find these sorts of people in a dance class, where they are completely free to wiggle and move as they like.

We all have a friend or family member who we would love to introduce to the benefits of yoga, who we know deep down, would never come. If you've ever asked yourself why, then perhaps this Reflex is the answer.

This is the Reflex of the wigglers and agitators who cannot keep still either in body or mind. The thought of having to sit still is torture so, at best if persuaded, may come to a more Vinyasa style class but will even hate the 2-minute relaxation at the end. Having their backs against the floor will trigger this Reflex and make them agitated again. Sometimes you will see a foot or hand tapping and eyes are open during Relaxation, as they try to contain the rising irritation at having to hold themselves still, as their whole body wants to move!

Children are prone to hold on to this Reflex and the children who are triggered by quiet and stillness, or who then fly off the wall (and barge into them sometimes) will be displaying this Reflex too.

The Spinal Galant is an important Reflex for those of us who have twitchy legs or are always tripping up over our own feet. It is important for those of us who are likely to get lost in our own thoughts and not be able to bring our attention to a single point.

If the thought of hours of stillness makes you very agitated, then this is also your Reflex. To some extent we all have it and the integration of this Reflex will help all of us. We will naturally feel calmer and more still in ourselves.

I enjoy working with children on this Reflex, as often they are getting into trouble at school or other activities for not being able to pay attention and 'stay still whilst listening'. There's very little understanding that for children with an active Spinal Galant, being still and taking in information is too difficult. They need the movement to be able to attend. Calming this Reflex down will help them to become more still and still be able to pay attention, meaning they will no longer be excluded, as is often the case, from the classroom.

I have always loved having my back stroked or scrubbed in the bath. Now I know why! The feedback it gives me helps to settle down any agitation I feel and so I can sleep better or relax more in the bath. I have great comfort in feeling into my back, it helps me to relax fully. And I can't imagine what it must be like for those of us who struggle to feel their backs, or when they do, are activated into agitation. Working on this Reflex for me, brings great comfort and I hope it will to you, if you need it to.

We have covered already that movement itself drives our development. From the very early stages of infanthood, throughout childhood and all the way into adulthood, we are making strong connections through the cerebellum. The cerebellum is important, as it feeds other areas of the brain and it regulates our movement, and our emotions and behaviour. If the cerebellum is not working smoothly, we will see difficulties in our rhythmic rocking. Rocking will not feel smooth and effortless, rather joltier.

The Spinal Galant Reflex influences how comfortably we sit, stand and walk. It helps us to exit the birth canal as we wiggle our way down, assists us in our early creeping and crawling and has an input into our vestibular (balance) centre development. It is an integral part of the preparation to develop our motor coordination and so helps to develop our strength in our lower back, pelvis and legs. This is why, when this Reflex is active, there is often a difficulty in walking and running and so all sports are generally avoided.

When given an option, lying down is preferred during activities (did you prefer to do your homework on the floor, for example?).

You will also see a child unable to sit back on a chair – the chair back irritates them, triggering the Reflex, so they would rather sprawl across the table if they cannot lie down!

There may also be a fixation or rigidity in the spine which makes coordination between the upper and lower body difficult. You often see this in swimming lessons; a child may be able to kick or do the arm strokes but when both are tried together, they sink!

The Spinal Galant is both a Primitive and a Transitional Reflex (bridging with the ATNR), and as such can make transitions difficult and unwelcome. Transitions are what power us through life and through the developmental arc itself. When there are changes in life, as simple as going from one room to another, or more complex, such as moving house, a retained Spinal Galant can lead to a whole host of new behaviour from poor focus to bed wetting.

This Reflex really affects our tactile sense (our sense of touch) and so touch may trigger it. You will find those of us who struggle with certain texture of clothes, labels or tight bands, can be triggered into survival mode. This is why someone with this Reflex will often wear loose clothing and trousers that fall down a lot! If our clothing is too tight, we cannot concentrate, follow written or verbal instruction and find trying to learn something new impossible.

Our interoception sense (our internal feeling world) is also developed through this Reflex, meaning that our ability to process feeling, and our subtle sensations and body vibrations depend on the good integration of this Reflex. If this is not the case, this can lead to difficulties in understanding how we feel and so we are unable to express or name our emotions. It also releases feelings of frustration and irritation when triggered, and we become impatient easily.

We may find touch irritating and tickly, making intimacy difficult. We may be more impulsive and struggle to settle down to anything, including sleep.

We may make impulsive decisions/responses that we then later regret. Saying things without thinking, perhaps brutally or irritatingly. When this is done too many times, we become insecure in our interactions and so have difficulty communicating, making decisions (we don't trust our judgement) or being happy with the decisions we have made. When emotions do come up, we have difficulty facing them – they are often overwhelming and so we'd rather avoid them altogether.

You know this Reflex is still active when you touch the area next to the spine on either side of the waist and the hips automatically swivel towards the point it has been touched. If this is retained, we see the muscles 'armour' where we contract the respiratory muscles and diaphragm and flex our legs, especially when repressing anxiety and anger. It also means that suddenly, when working on this Reflex, we realise we need to use the loo. Not only because we feel the need but because stimulation of the lower spine will activate the Reflex, causing the need to urinate. This is why a child will be continuing to wet the bed after age 5.

A retained Spinal Galant can also lead to the activation of the Tendon Guard Reflex which protects the tendons and muscles in the legs. The calf muscles shorten, the knees bend and lock and the body rises up on the toes (tiptoe walking). At the same time we see the muscles of the back and neck contracts.

When we have worked on this Reflex and it begins to integrate, we see better communication, speech and language, particularly our emotional intelligence in adults. We will be less tetchy and intolerant, meaning we have better relationships too.

We will also have better focus and awareness, being able to

access the still inner state and grow our mental discipline. This makes mindfulness and meditation accessible with all the wisdom and inner connection it brings.

Our confidence builds as we trust and know ourselves better, our anxiety lessens, and we have more drive to achieve our dreams. Most importantly, we are able to fully relax and sleep better! Our whole body will feel more settled when we are still.

PERSONAL PRACTICE

Before you begin your practice for the Spinal Galant Reflex, bring yourself to have a sense into your back and its position. Can you feel all of your back? Are you able to divide your back up into sections (top right shoulder blade, bottom left pelvis area, top left shoulder blade, bottom right pelvis area)? How do you feel if you imagine someone were to poke you in the back right now? Are you ticklish? If someone told you that you had to sit completely still for an hour, how would you react?

Spend some time thinking over the responses and then do the practice on the video.

Please feel free to visit **www.the-empowered-feminine.co.uk** for a Spinal Galant-based yoga practice example. At the end of this book there are details of how to access the videos that accompany this book.

www.the-empowered-feminine.co.uk

Now how does your back feel at the end of the practice? How does it feel when you are lying down after relaxation? If someone were to touch your back, how would you react? How has the feeling in your back affected the rest of your body? Now if you were asked to be still for a long while, would it feel more possible?

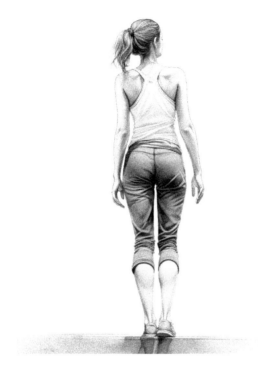

MOVEMENTS AND EXERCISES FOR INTEGRATING THE SPINAL GALANT

Back Stroking

Bring both your hands to your lower back and give your back a rub. See how sensitive or numb it is. Give this a number on a scale of 0-10. Zero being completely numb, and 10 overwhelmingly sensitive.

Now with only one hand, stroke down from as high up as you can reach towards your buttock, then swap and do the alternate side. (If you can find someone to help, get them to start at shoulder level.)

Now begin to stroke in a rhythmic manner until you feel you have had enough or until 2 minutes have passed.

Feel into your back now, without touching it, how does it feel on a scale of 0-10?

Cat-Cow

Bring yourself onto all fours and check to make sure your hands and knees are directly below your shoulder and hip joints. Imagine that on your back are four hotplates, like on a cooker and begin to move the base of the spine, make sure that both lower hotplates start to move simultaneously and that as you move the spine upwards the two upper hotplates move together.

Ask yourself if you are putting equal push through both hotplates, then begin the reverse movement in the tail and do the same as above. If you have difficulty identifying your four hotplates, ask someone to rub these areas, as above, for a couple of minutes so you can feel them.

Pelvic Eight Exercises

This movement can be done cross-legged or on all fours. Sitting in a cross-legged position, begin to move the pelvis in a circular motion until you feel the circles very much in your awareness. Then begin to move in a figure of eight motion. Initially it may be easier to start standing up and move into a sitting position after you have managed a figure of eight movement on your feet. You can also try this on all fours.

As above, bring yourself onto all fours with your hands directly beneath your shoulders and your knees directly beneath your hips. Imagine once again you have four hotplates on your back. It may help to have someone rub those four hotplates again so you can feel them more clearly.

Once you have mastered the figure of eight movement in one direction, see if you can do it going the other way. Experiment, trying it faster and slower, work out which speed and rhythm you prefer.

WHAT TO DO IF YOU FEEL YOU ARE SPINAL GALANT TRIGGERED

As we work our way up the developmental arc, we may find that there is one Reflex that can make us feel a little spaced out or brain foggy, or triggered at worst. If your system does become overwhelmed with this Reflex, you may experience body disorientation, an urgent need to go to the toilet, or an unusual surge of intolerance or irritability. If you continue regardless of these signs, you may feel lower abdominal pain, red ears, nausea, backache or creeping anxiety. As before, do in the first instance, listen to your body carefully, so you can catch the milder signs of overwhelm and as soon as you realise, implement the Feet, Hands and Face Reflex. Spend some time really feeling into the FHF until the nervous system calms down.

OTHER EXERCISES FOR SPINAL GALANT INTEGRATION

Raising Awareness in the Spinal Galant Relaxation

Ask yourself if you would rather lie on your back or your front for relaxation. When you have chosen your preferred position, bring your awareness to your right hand and fingers. Feel all five fingers and the hand, and work your attention up the arm, through the elbow and the shoulder to where in your back you feel the arm is joined. It will be somewhere in your upper right hand shoulder area (The upper right 'hotplate').

Now bring your awareness to your left hand and fingers. Feel all five fingers and the hand and work your attention up the arm through the elbow and the shoulder to where in your back you feel the arm is joined. It will be somewhere in your upper left hand shoulder area. (The upper left 'hotplate').

Now bring your awareness to your right foot and toes. Feel all the toes and your foot and work your way up the leg; feeling the calves, shins, knees and up the thigh, until you can feel roughly where the leg is attached into your back (the lower right 'hotplate').

Next feel all the toes and your foot on the left and work your way up the leg, feeling the calves, shins, knees and up the thigh until you can feel roughly where the leg is attached into your back (the lower left 'hotplate').

Bring your awareness now to all four limbs and where they connect into the back and find a way to help the back relax even more. Perhaps imagining you are lying on a memory foam mattress that sinks a little as you relax, or that you are made of wax, and you are slowly melting into the floor.

AFFIRMATIONS:

'I may feel restless or irritable. However, I know I am safe and calm in the world.'

'I accept all my wriggles and love myself still.'

'My body is quiet and still.'

'I heal as I relax.'

'I am relaxing; I am relaxed.'

OTHER ACTIVITIES FOR SPINAL GALANT INTEGRATION:

- Back massages
- Hot stone massage
- Acupressure mat
- In swimming, backstroke

YOGA WITH THE SPINAL GALLANT INTEGRATED

Now that you have so much more awareness of your back, you can begin to feel into how your body (and your back) moves. Raising awareness in the back helps us enormously with the two Reflexes that follow, the STNR and the ATNR. It is important for our future ability to connect more complex parts of our neurology and body. Use these following exercises after raising awareness in the back to further integrate what you have learnt.

This Reflex brings good awareness of the 3D alignment of the body. You will be able to feel all four 'hotplates,' and what position they are always in, making it easier to understand where your body is in space depending on what asana you are practicing. Giving yourself the correct commands for example, in a side bend, is my hip down, my shoulder up? Has my hip moved forward or is it aligned with my shoulder?

Cross Crawl

Now that we have these four areas nicely grounded, bring yourself onto all fours and feel the four 'hotplates' on your back, now begin to cross crawl. Another alternative is to lie on our back on the floor, always keeping these four areas in contact with the floor and then cross crawl.

Leg Raises

If there is a lot of tension in the lower back and legs, a raised leg stretching sequence is also a good thing to do. Raise one leg at a time and ground the lower two 'hotplates' into the floor evenly. For a sciatic stretch, the leg can also be allowed to fall to the side but without the 'hotplates' lifting off the floor.

Forward Bend

When standing, you can bring your attention to the four areas of the hotplates. Now, as your arms come up over your head to stretch, feel the two upper 'hotplates' stretch evenly and keep them aligned as you forward bend, ensuring the lower two hotplates stay inline too.

Triangle Poses

In Triangle Poses, it is easy for the pelvis to come out of alignment and for the shoulders to rotate out of alignment. Bring your feet as far apart as you comfortably can so that you are in Triangle Pose. As you do a Triangle Forward Bend Pose, be aware of the tension felt and the urge to come out of alignment. If you feel you are coming out of alignment (one hotplate moving forward and another moving back for example), align yourself as best you can, using a slight push through the legs as needed.

Half Cobra Forward Bend

Sitting on the floor with one leg straight, one leg bent, check whether or not the bottom two 'hotplates' are aligned and if not, move your pelvis accordingly. As you forward bend, check that your shoulders are also in line, so that all four hotplates form an even rectangle.

Side Bends

Sitting with legs wide, allow the body to bend forwards and then rotate towards one of the feet. Be aware of the four 'hotplates' staying aligned. It is easy in this pose for either the shoulder or the hip to move forward or back.

CASE STUDIES

I have worked with many children who are being excluded a lot from mainstream learning because they do not move or become still like other children. In one school, where the way they teach is not mainstream, parents are even advised that perhaps this type of school is not for their child because they aren't 'moving with the flock'.

This was the case with P. He is 6 years old and already labelled a bit of a troublemaker though the teacher refers to it in a more disguised way saying, 'He's very lively!' He is however often out of the main room of play and learning and on his own with a helper, waiting to be calmed down. There is absolutely nothing else the teacher has issue with, other than he doesn't join in with the activities when asked to. And when brought over (not by force, but you get my meaning, by 'encouragement of the strongest kind'), he isn't exactly happy to participate!

Luckily for P, his mum is a psychiatrist who works with children all the time and she could see that there wasn't anything in particular wrong with her boy. Instead, when she heard about the Primitive Reflexes, she did her research and came to me for treatment. I see them about once a month as she is very good at implementing all the exercises and yoga practices herself. Needless to say, within in a year, P is no problem at all and is happily ready to begin more formal learning as he moves up the school year.

SPINAL GALANT IN YOGA PRACTICE

The Spinal Galant is one of the Reflexes where you will begin to learn much more about body management. It seems also to be a bit more common in the general population. It is advisable to go easy at first with the integration exercises, perhaps only doing one or two at a time. And reminding yourself regularly to keep checking for yourself if there are any symptoms of 'overdoing it,' as this is more likely.

Pause for as long as you need to, and to do no more integration, if you feel any of the following: heat in the face, ears or body, nausea, excessive yawning, wild thoughts and any kind of discomfort. With children it is easier, as they will tell you one way or another if they have had enough. But adults, especially in a yoga class situation, will want to 'keep up' and will override the warnings.

Having said all this, it is also the one Reflex where most people really feel a difference – whether it's 'their' Reflex or not, and is very useful for us, as it helps enormously in describing how to do an asana to ourselves.

There are different focuses that you can have at any given time, here follow some examples:

METHOD 1 – HOTPLATE GROUNDING AWARENESS

Having worked through the hotplate sequence, you should be able to feel, when you are on your back, all four areas (hotplates) in contact with the ground and feel supported by the ground. Here, it is useful to use this support to stretch and cement this feeling.

Lift one leg up into the air and feel the weight of it sink into the corresponding 'hotplate'. Then lift the other leg; feel that supported and sinking into the floor and then do the same with the arms. You will finish with all four limbs in the air feeling grounded through the four hotplates.

With this support in place, it is now easy to begin some movement. For example, you can bring in the knees towards the chest and stretch the back and feel how the four 'hotplates' support the stretch. Once you have felt this, bring your legs and arms back down to the ground and continue to feel this support even though the legs and arms are on the floor. From here, there are a variety of asanas that can be used with this grounding technique in mind.

For example, the Bridge Pose:

Bring the soles of the feet onto the floor and feel the four 'hotplates' sink into the ground. As the tail tucks in between the legs, see if you can still feel the four areas grounded.

Engaging the core, begin pushing through the feet to feel the weight shift onto the top two 'hotplates. Allow the body to melt into these top two 'hotplates' but be aware, as you come down to feel the lower two 'hotplates' again take the weight of the body.

Other poses where this method works well are:

Shoulder Stands

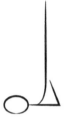

Happy Baby Pose

Wind Relieving Pose

Any pose/sequence that is lying on your back.

METHOD 2 – USING LOWER BACK WARMTH

Another method that is nice to use after the back rubbing integration exercise, is to bring awareness to the warmth in the lower two 'hotplates' of the back to bring a greater sense of upper and lower body. Keeping an awareness of the (literally) hot lower two hotplates, as you perform the asanas, will keep the lower back more relaxed as well, and will aid in letting go of tension. This ties in well with the FPR and Landau Reflex too.

Remember or feel the heat/tingle/whatever you felt in your back. (If you've just done the integration exercise, this really helps). Now ground this heat into the floor either through the legs and feet (if standing) or through the bottom (if sitting) or through the floor (if lying down). It can feel different for different people so perhaps you feel the heat, coming from the lower two 'hotplates' down into the legs and floor. Now keeping this feeling in mind, lift the top two hotplates and create space between them. Stretch the space between the upper and lower two hotplates away from each other and at the same time relaxing the lower two 'hotplates' with the feeling of heat or tingle.

For example, in Seated Forward Fold:

Feel the heat in the lower two 'hotplates' which have just been rubbed and allow them to sink into the floor whilst the legs relax (FPR Reflex). Then as you lift up your arms, feel the top two 'hotplates' move away from the lower two 'relaxing' ones. Keep this relaxing, warm, sinking feeling in the lower two 'hotplates,' as the upper two stretch up and over towards the legs as you fold forwards. Using the breath, you can feel the lower two 'plates' sink and relax as the top two lift with each in-breath.

Other poses where this method works well are:

Hero Pose

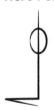

Chair Pose

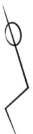

Standing Forward Bend

Downward Dog

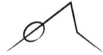

CONCLUSION

I often try to imagine what it must be like to live with this Reflex. How keeping still would be difficult and finding the inner calm I am so familiar with almost impossible. I imagine myself trying to meditate and almost getting to a place of focused awareness, only to have it cruelly snatched away from me by the sensations in my body of agitation and the need for constant movement. I'm sure I would soon begin to think there was something wrong with me, that I cannot simply attend to something for a while, like all those around me seem able to. My self-worth would slowly begin to be eroded as I try and try again only to be let down. Soon I would believe that 'I simply can't' focus.

The lack of focus itself would make life difficult too. Unable to complete tasks and to follow through on my own personal desires would lead me to a place where I'd begin to believe I was useless and not capable. You can begin to see how it is that the inner voices in someone's head would grow and grow until you were full of voices telling you how terrible you are at everything.

When the body finally can be still, after working with this Reflex, we are finally centred and grounded and home. From this place of stillness, we can start to see that we are entitled to go after what we want, that we deserve it. Our self-worth increases and we begin to take the steps towards fulfilling our dreams and not finding ourselves distracted by what is not important. Knowing our destination and seeing the steps towards it, we can ask for help and support and feel worthy of that support because now we feel we can fulfil our aims. We won't be letting anyone down, including ourselves.

LITTLE BIRD

I bleed for you, dear Sister,
Little Bird carrying your broken wing.
You have stepped into the Vipers Nest
And hypnotised, you are sinking into his coils.

Soon you shall be knotted, trapped, just like I was.

Except that I have awoken,
Stepped out of the dream.
For it was a deception of the illusionary kind
That kept me there for so long.
The lie that was love,
When there was only possession.

I bleed for you, dear Sister,
Little Bird with your broken wing.
For it took a gargantuan effort for me to be free
Yet you have stepped straight into my hollow in the nest.

Here you will suffer at the hands of snakes, just as I did.

Except that I have warned you,
And when the coils feel too tight, you will remember;
For it is real, what I have learned
And the illusion is now gone.

The sad resemblance of love
When there was so much more out there to be had.

I bleed for you, dear Sister,
Little bird, nurse your broken wings,
For you need them to learn to fly high.
Let the illusion break for a moment.

And fly, fly, fly for the hills, just as I did.

Veronika Peña de la Jara

CHAPTER 6

Symbiotic Tonic Neck Reflex (STNR)

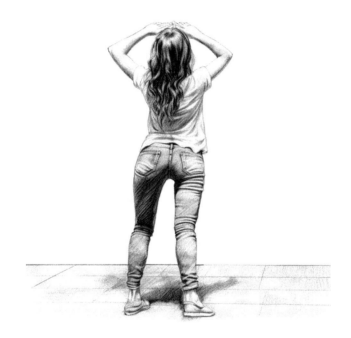

The Symbiotic Tonic Neck Reflex (STNR) comes up regularly in my yoga classes, as it is one of the Reflexes that deals with naturally setting up posture, ensuring good core control and over all body strength. These are some of the reasons many people come to yoga class in the first place, of course. For a lot of people, yoga is about having good posture, and this is the Reflex that achieves this. In modern times, we find that doctors, for example, will refer people with bad backs to contemporary yoga and Pilates to 'strengthen' or 'become free of compression'.

What I love about this Reflex, is that it comes so easily to most people and most practitioners will be able to feel an immediate difference within a few integration exercises. There is so much joy when you realise that there is something happening to you, that it isn't your failure 'to stay upright' that is causing you problems. Here is help of the automatic kind that you can harness, initially with some effort, which then has the potential to work all by itself and become automatic.

This immediacy really opens our minds to the power of the Reflex work and how it 'wakes up' the neural networks in the spine. At the end of a yoga session using this Reflex, you are much more aware of your posture and the actual shape of your spine, but also how natural it is to hold it upright. Most of us struggle to hold our spine up and are often in tension to keep it upright. We are used to putting in conscious awareness into our posture. What if we could have good posture without even thinking about it?

It is rare to see young babies sitting in a slouched position. Most babies are beautifully upright without any effort whatsoever. So we know that it is possible for us as adults to have this ease of posture too. There are all sorts of reasons as to why our posture may well have become strained, and this Reflex helps us to come back to that original pattern of uprightness we had as young babies.

There is a lot of pressure in our society to look good, to be healthy and to be capable, and nothing shows it more if we are failing, than our posture. We then feel pressured into sorting it out ourselves, or we hide from it feeling guilty and are disappointed at the amount of effort it takes or at our absolute failure to achieve it. When you understand that so much of our system is not under our immediate control, there is the freedom to work which allows us the time and space to reach our goal without pressure and with faith in the outcome.

My STNR Reflex was affected in two ways by the fact that I was still holding the Moro Reflex. When I sat to meditate, for example, I would always notice after a while that I was sticking my tail out and lifting my chin (in an S position). I would attempt to bring myself into a more neutral spine position, only to lose concentration and find myself back in an S position again. This little fight, caused by my tendency to drop my breastbone due to diaphragmatic tightness, was also due to a weak core after having 3 children. Staying with a neutral spine, requires a core! Having meditated for long periods over 25 years, I can now safely say that I can activate my core and sit for an hour or so without moving much, keeping my spine straight without any effort. Knowing where 'straight' is, has been part of this journey for me.

Having this pillar of support within me had helped me to be more emotionally stable. When difficult situations are presented to me, I no longer run off and hide. Instead, I feel myself become more upright, draw on my inner strength, take a breath and consider my response, if I do respond at all. I can centre myself as needed, and work from there, deciding what the best outcome is for me. This could be to walk away, but it could also be to say what needs to be said. Now the choice is mine to make.

Having the full support of the spine throughout life cannot be underestimated. I can imagine what it must be like if you are in constant pain or if your backbone does not respond to you, how hard life must become. Our spine gives us a sense of internal support, of being strong and ready for the world.

Whenever I have had back pain, the overall feelings have always been of not being able to cope with day-to-day life. Everything feels too much and there is resistance to doing anything that may take me over my 'limit'. Having a straight, yet comfortable inner support system makes you feel like you can move through life with ease – everything is possible. You can begin to believe and trust in yourself and your reasons for being here in the world. You begin to explore your purpose, your reasons for existing and what you may have to contribute to those around you and to the world.

The Core work also helps you to become more aware of your 'centre' a term that took me years to understand. The Core feels like the control centre of all my body movement now. For a long time, this had been non-existent, giving me a feeling of 'floating' through life.

The spine is also connecting your entire body into one efficient moving whole. You begin to feel like a whole human being, not blown up into tiny fragments like when you are in survival mode. This feeling of centre and wholeness will feed into feelings of being both connected to the earthly realm and also the emotional and spiritual body, the 'inner self' or 'being'. There is a sense of being fully integrated into a whole human being when your posture fully supports your body. So much so, that we can trust our spine to hold us and so we can also begin to feel we can trust life to hold us too. And in this deeper knowing of being held, we open the door perhaps to something bigger than us.

I often equate it to the feeling you get when you come across a huge tree that has been standing for hundreds of years. This tree is part of a massive eco-system which it does not question – it just is. There is a sense of quiet strength and support for all the wildlife around it and within it. It lives immersed in it. And it's all done in such an unassuming way. This sense brings us closer to being connected to the nature of things and to open our minds to questions like, 'What part do we play in our own ecosystem?' 'What is the source of all life'? 'How can such a small acorn, produce such a huge oak tree?' Whatever our beliefs, we become closer to the source of all things and all life.

Although we have looked so far mainly at the STNR in relation to the spine, it is also setting up the upper and lower body to work together and make the connections we need for crawling and walking. We are gaining the body control and hand-eye motor skills for other activities like swimming and tennis and other sports.

The STNR is important for our neurological make up as it is making connections from the brainstem (primitive brain) through the limbic (emotional brain) to the prefrontal cortex (executive, modern brain).

This Reflex is making connections into the pineal gland which is located in the middle of our brains at the level of our eyes and can help us to connect to our cognitive experiences of a spiritual kind. The pineal is a portal of growth into insight, inner vision and self-definition. The pineal also has a very important role in the release of melatonin, which affects our ability to sleep and rest deeply. It manages our circadian rhythms, including signals that make us feel tired, sleep, wake up and be alert at the same time each day. Melatonin is produced in the pineal according to the amount of light a person is exposed to. When it darkens melatonin increases. The pineal activates during meditation and its relationship with the circadian rhythms may indicate why dawn is the best time to meditate.

Serotonin, the neurotransmitter (happy chemical) responsible for your mood, is transformed into melatonin in the pineal gland. A decline in melatonin in the body triggers the aging process in our bodies too, so we can see how important the pineal gland is to our body. However, it is also widely researched that the pineal gland is the key to our spiritual awakening.

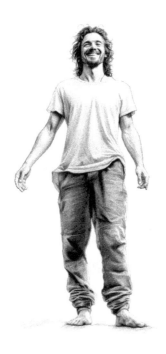

INTEGRATING THE STNR

When the STNR first arrives in our developmental arc, its initial job is to help us to crawl. It then sticks around to help us achieve good posture and good upper and lower body control. First though, we need to go from sitting to all fours and it is in these movements that we see the STNR Integration exercises emerge. The STNR movements also will enable the head to be able to move independently of the body. The arms and legs are no longer dependent on the position of our head, and we can make a distinction between the spine working as a unit or working our upper and lower spine. We are setting up our patterning of strong upper body strength, proper posture and tone in the back and the neck. We gain more proprioceptive understanding and can organise left and right, up and down, front and back, above and below.

If this Reflex is not well integrated, we may see the spine moving as one-unit, upper body weakness and bad posture. You may not be able to coordinate breaststroke in swimming lessons, you may find yourself slumping when you sit, and your shoulders may be hunched when you aren't paying attention. Children may sit in a 'W' position or may wrap their legs around chairs to keep themselves upright, they may lie over their books when doing homework at a table for example.

If this Reflex is retained, there will be a miscommunication between the primitive brain (basal ganglia) and the prefrontal cortex. This could lead to problems with focusing at far and near distances making ball games impossible. Arm strength will be compromised and the monkey bars in a playground cannot be climbed, push ups and somersaults difficult to achieve. This Reflex also affects the heart and the heart rate, so you may be more disinclined to want to exercise, if your lack of strength hasn't already put you off! The breath may feel obstructed and uncomfortable.

With there being insufficient stimulation to the prefrontal cortex, we may also experience problems with attention and concentration. This is why this Reflex is closely linked to learning and learning development. It interferes with good posture for reading and writing, for example. It significantly affects penmanship as you will be using your entire body (including neck and legs) making the process exhausting.

If you are identifying with this Reflex, you may well have not crawled as a child or had difficulties sitting at a table or desk. You would have hated ball games and had other difficulties with sports that require upper and lower body coordination. Sitting for longer periods of time would have led to problems with attention and therefore access to learning. There may well have been sleep issues and poor impulse control.

As an adult, you may experience low muscle tone and have bad posture. You probably hate strong exercise! You may be more comfortable sitting with your legs up or with your legs crossed. You may have difficulties sleeping and perhaps you have difficulties meditating too.

In more extreme cases, you may have a rigid, fixed spine, alongside a more rigid way of being. There may be poor impulse control perhaps extending into obsessive compulsive disorders. You may have upper and lower body disassociation and visual or spatial processing difficulties. There may be an irregular heart rhythm and shallow breathing.

MOVEMENTS TO INTEGRATE THE STNR

Before you begin your STNR movement session, have a go at this exercises and then repeat it at the end to see if you can feel the difference. On hands and knees try to do a push up on the floor. How hard is it, how much work are you doing? How many can you do before you are tired? Sitting on the floor, check in with your spine. How straight is it? Can you feel any tension anywhere holding yourself upright? Breathe out and feel if your core is working. Can you feel it at all? Now continue to do the integrative exercises.

Cross-Legged Push-Pull

Sitting cross-legged on the floor, bring your hands onto the floor in front of you and lookup. Repeat a few times. After a few times, as you put the hands on the floor, also push slightly and feel the effect on the upper back and chest area and the spine, going from S shape to C shape and back a few times. Make sure that the hands are managing the movement, not the back.

Bouncing on Knees

Sit on the floor with your knees bent and your legs tucked under you in a kneeling position. Now swing the body forward and land your hands on the floor and then lookup. Now push yourself back towards the heels again, looking down. Initially, this may feel a little uncoordinated, with the head coming to look up or down after the body has moved.

Repeat the movement slowly until everything is happening at once. Landing on your hands and looking up. Landing on your heels and looking down. When this is more fluid repeat a few times until you can do it in a bouncing rhythm.

Somersault Rolls

Again, sit on the floor with your legs tucked beneath you in a kneeling position. Now bring your hands on the floor but this time bring the head to the floor between your hands. Let your hands support the head a little bit so not all your body weight is on your neck and head. When you feel confident begin to roll slightly over the top of your head. Then push yourself back onto your heels again. Keep working backwards and forwards between having the top of your head on the floor and the forehead on the floor. Repeat as many times as feels comfortable.

Cat-Cow

Place yourself on the floor on all fours. Leading by the tailbone as you breathe in, move your tail upwards and look up, your back will arch in an 'S' shape as your tummy moves towards the floor.

Next as you breathe out, the tailbone begins to move towards pointing down to the floor, your back arches up and head curls in. You are now trying to point the eyes towards your pubic bone, and you are in 'C' shape.

Now sit again crossed-legged on the floor. What is the first thing you notice about your spine? Are you straighter, how much effort is there?

Do another push up on your hands and knees. Does it feel easier? How many can you do before you feel tired? Can you feel the difference from earlier?

OTHER EXERCISES FOR INTEGRATING THE STNR

Raising Spine and Pineal Awareness

Using as many cushions and bolsters as you need, get into a comfortable child's pose. Take the time to get comfortable in this position. Once in position, focus on feeling your breath push against the cushions or thighs as you breathe in and as you breathe out.

Now begin to focus on how your breathing is moving up and down your spine. Really feel the breath travel up and down the spine. Feel how connected you are to your spine, how well you can feel it.

Next, sit up in a cross-legged position and close your eyes. Bring your eyes to point up towards your pineal gland between your eyes and focus on any sensations that you may begin to have as you observe this space. Be aware of the rhythm of your breath.

AFFIRMATIONS:

"I am present, I am here, I am now."

"I sit strong and long."

"I know who I am."

"I can feel my inner self."

"I have landed in me."

OTHER ACTIVITIES FOR INTEGRATING STNR:

- Spend time in the sunlight every day.
- Sleep in complete darkness.
- Commit to a regular meditation practice, as this will develop and enhance your pineal gland.
- Yogic practices are very potent methods for awakening the pineal gland. Inversions are particularly helpful as they increase blood flow to the pineal while you are upside down.
- The practice of Yoga Nidra or yogic sleep meditation also helps to awaken the pineal gland.

CASE STUDY

One of my favourite classes is teaching Reflex Yoga to horse riders. I have two groups, one for disabilities and one for jockeys. In both groups, posture is important to them and finding out that it isn't an automatic 'fault' of theirs that causes your posture to be slightly off is liberating. As I understand it, a lot of time is spent learning to ride and of this plenty is spent on posture.

As we shall have seen, good posture is not necessarily automatic for many people for all sorts of reasons. Having a good few Reflex exercises and yoga classes to reinforce what you are learning has helped many horse riders I have known. Notable examples are in those with disabilities. One case comes to mind. Can you imagine how hard it must be to stay balanced on a horse if you are not in full use of your legs?

My lovely student, M, was born without legs from the knee down and without full hands either. She usually gets around on a scooter, so the freedom of horse riding is her most happy place. She is a competent rider but struggles to be on a horse for long as it causes so much strain on her hips, particularly as she is using them to hold on, literally! The harness she has makes it unnecessary to do so but her survival instinct is to 'hold on!' Although young M is having to limit her riding time, and of course, it doesn't bode well for her hips in the future.

There is also the added complication that there is hypermobility in her joints. Being more upright will help with relaxing her legs into position, as she will feel much more balanced (currently she leans forward, sticking out her tail). And so the work she is learning in our classes is helping her to be more relaxed and upright at the same time. Although new to my classes, in the few weeks we have been working, already there is less pain after riding sessions.

STNR IN YOGA PRACTICE

The STNR is a great Reflex to work with, as it is full of energy and will power and helps us to feel motivated and connected to ourselves. Often, we arrive at a yoga session feeling weary and tired, and wishing we had more to inspire us in life. The STNR is a great Reflex to inspire us and to keep us coming back to yoga for more.

It is of course, also important for posture. As one of the main postural set of Reflexes, this Reflex, alongside the Landau and Tonic Labyrinthic Neck Reflex (TLR) can really revolutionise how you can feel upright, straight and strong.

The STNR can bring smoother function between upper and lower body, so it is good for all those poses that are a little harder to manage. It is also excellent for learning core engagement which is very much needed by most of the post-partum population. If you wish to tackle something a little more challenging, this is a good Reflex to work with.

Do keep a lookout though that you are not struggling with anything a little harder, and give yourself easier alternatives if necessary. I always find that starting with the easier options is better. Then introduce the variations that may be more challenging, not the other way around. The competitive nature of humans will always try for the harder variations. So remember, it is an option and not for everyone.

METHOD 1 – FROM GROSS TO SUBTLE

With this method, we begin our practice by integrating the STNR exercises using the 'bigger' movement types, like the Cat-Cow. Having done some asanas to complement this integration, we then do some more subtle integration exercises, like observing our breath as it moves up and down the spine. Then we do more asanas to help these more subtle movements. We begin by noticing how we move from 'S' to 'C' just as we breathe in and breathe out and then bring this to asanas that are a little more static, so that students can feel it for themselves.

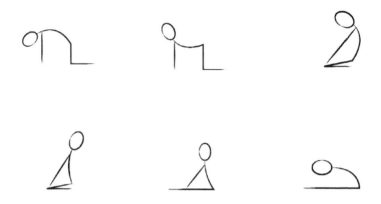

For example: Start with Cat-Cow and move on to Forward Bend

Once again place yourself on the floor on all fours and, as explained above, begin your practice with a Cat-Cow. Leading by the tailbone as you breathe in, move your tail upwards and look up, your back will arch in an 'S' shape as your tummy moves towards the floor.

Now as you breathe out, the tailbone begins to move towards pointing down to the floor, your back arches up and head curls in. You are now trying to point the eyes towards your pubic bone, and you are in 'C' shape.

Next sit on the floor with your legs out in front of you. Reach forward as far as is comfortable, but you can still feel a stretch in your hamstrings and back, all the way to your neck.
Without moving, begin to breathe, and remember how, when you breathe in, the spine arched a little into an S shape and how, when you breathed out it moved a little into a C shape. If you cannot feel the subtlety of the movement while you are still, try a baby version of the S to C movement and then try again with no movement.

Other asanas that work well with this method are:

Downward Dog

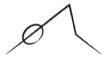

All Standing Forward Bends

Twists

Standing Triangle Forward Bend

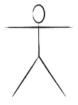

All Side Bends

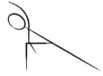

This method works well with yoga sequences as well. Think about the combination of asanas that work well in large movements of the spine going forward and back. Sun Salutation, Swan and the Hindi Press-up, for example.

METHOD 2 – AWARENESS OF STRAIGHT SPINE

Whilst integrating the STNR exercises, do a 'before' and 'after' awareness of the spine exercise, so that you can feel the difference in your own body.

Sit up as comfortably as you can, without doing anything specifically to your spine. Now in your mind's eye, go through your spine, starting at the bottom and working your way up. And have a sense of the shape of it. Perhaps draw it in your mind.

Now do a few of the STNR integration exercises and have a look at the spine again. Does it feel different? What has changed? Where exactly has it straightened out?

Now challenge yourself with some asanas that have the potential to pull you out of straightness if that awareness is not there.

For example: Chair Pose

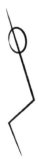

In standing position, allow your knees to bend, as you bring your arms above your head. Imagine that you are about to sit on a chair. Keep bending your knees and hold the position as you feel into your spine.

As you move your arms up above your head, how does the spine change shape? Can you keep the spine still or does it have to move? Can you isolate the movement so that only your shoulders are rotating? Do you feel a holding in your lower back (FPR) or a collapsing in your breastbone (Moro)? What position have you moved your head into (TLR)?

Other poses that work well for this method are:

Standing Table Pose

Downward Dog

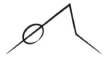

Shoulder Stand

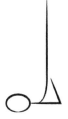

Sitting Forward Bend

METHOD 3 – ACTIVATING THE CORE

For this method, it may take a few tries to get the core 'feeling' right. Most people over-compensate for a lack of core, using their back muscles, even tightening their anus instead. It can be a long journey, especially after childbirth for women, to find our core again.

In this method, we will focus, at least to start with, on the C shape of the STNR moves. As you go through the integration exercises, pay attention to the Core area as you move into the C shape. You may begin to feel a little, natural pull upwards. It feels a little like you are sucking something up your vulva (for men the area between your anus and your ability to stop pee, the perineum). It may be out of your reach of feeling to begin with, as it is so subtle. So I would suggest you practice this feeling in a couple of stronger poses.

For Example, Swing and Balance Poses

The Swing

Sitting cross-legged (or straight-legged, though it is harder) on the floor, make your spine into a C shape and bring your hands level with your mid-thigh. It is important that your hands aren't too far back, or you will compensate and use your upper body instead.

Now gently begin to imagine that your arms are the poles of a swing and try to lift the swing seat by using your Core. You may find it goes nowhere! Yet you will feel a sense of 'picking up,' 'sucking up' or 'closing' in the inner core area. Keep practicing this over and over until it is a familiar feeling.

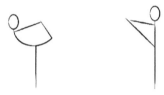

Balance Poses

Once you have established the area you are 'picking up' try some balance poses, even if you feel unsteady and must hold the wall or chair, the Core, now active will help.

This time, however, as you are standing up, you may also feel a pickup coming right down in the arches of your feet, up through the inner thighs and into the core area itself.

Start with something easy and work up to being able to hold your leg up out in front of you straight.

Other poses that work well with this method are:

Boat Pose

Bridge Pose

Side Floor Triangle

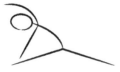

Shoulder Stand

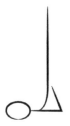

CONCLUSION

Having a straight, strong and present spine helps us to know who we are, what we 'stand' for and to be able to use the power of our centre 'core' to power us through life, so we can become who we were meant to be.

Once we are out of the Survival Reflexes that hold our spine locked in certain positions, we can flow through life with grace and poise. Free to move, our spine sits in a comfortable position, is naturally upright and we can build a sense of 'having a backbone' as the saying goes.

Having a core brings us into the awareness of our centre from which we distribute the lifeforce energy throughout our body. Traditionally in most bodywork exercises the core is the centre of this exchange. In conjunction with the Landau Reflex, the spine being free to move, allows us to reach better for our needs and for help when we need it as we strive to make something of ourselves. We are no longer surviving, now we are thriving.

I AM AN IMMIGRANT

I have been an immigrant all my life,
though neither by choice nor nature.
A fair-weather bird picked me unripe
from the family tree
and dropped me across many oceans
Upon hard sodden soil.

Miraculously, I have been growing all my life
Upon this hard foreign land.
I may have grown straight and tall,
had not the back door
guilty attentions, spontaneously
watered and fed me.

I may have been bent and crooked all my life,
my branches reaching for remembered sun, but I am not.
The forest of my infancy, it's sandy giving soil by sandy seas
Surrounded by those that knew me
and loved me well, remembered in my genes.

Somehow, I have produced seeds of my very own
Who fed upon this fertile soil
And grew tall and strong.
Amazingly, I must have had it in me;

For I grew broad, hollow, but strong
and together we made a home.

At some point, a fateful farmer gave me a hazel stake
A firm worthy support.
He too took root and blossomed,
Our roots now intertwined; our branches crossed,
The land of my home no longer called so.

Around us we have our own family forest;
Our saplings have flown.
The wrenching feeling of sunny climes
replaced by rains and rainbows bright.
Finally, I can leave behind that sunny coast –
After 40 years I truly reside.

Veronika Peña de la Jara

CHAPTER 7

Asymmetric Tonic Neck Reflex (ATNR)

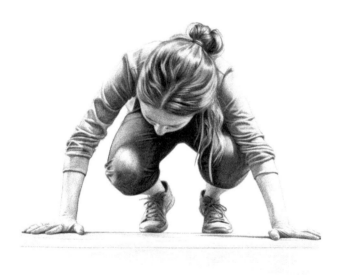

The Asymmetric Tonic Neck Reflex (ATNR) is a popular request in Reflex Yoga, as it helps enormously with the feeling of being present, connected and to be one's best self. When you think of those times that you feel 'foggy,' 'lost' and 'out of it,' it seems impossible that you might have a way to bring yourself back. Of course, we know that most yoga practice helps with this, as movement has an ability to reconnect us. The ATNR has a quality of connection that is beyond this, however, as you feel sharp, present and somehow whole.

This Reflex, for some people, can be difficult to grasp and the movements will take a lot of practice. It is easy to see improvements, however. Visually you begin to see the coordination, for example, become smoother and perhaps steadier and more enduring. On a more internal level, I have found that I am less forgetful, more organised and aware of time management. I use this Reflex a lot with my U3A (University of the Third Age) as it helps to keep the mind active better than playing chess or doing crosswords. It's the combination of brainwork with movement that makes it so powerful for this group.

Some of the movements have even been researched extensively enough in scientific research to prove that a rise in 30% IQ is possible. Imagine that! It means a lot, particularly for children who are struggling to learn, that here is something that can really help them. Many a time, faith has been restored in a child or teenager struggling to learn. It is not that they are stupid, as they have allowed themselves to believe, but that their connectivity needed some help. Nothing boosts morale more than knowing that something you thought was inevitable can be changed. It is a life lesson to all of us that we don't need to accept 'what we are' and can always find ways of learning and improving ourselves.

There is a lot of pressure in society to perform intellectually, which is often not available to those with a retained ATNR. As we will see later in this chapter, this particularly affects those with ADHD, ADD, dyslexia, and dyspraxia, who have learning difficulties. Work with these movements can absolutely make learning accessible to all these groups. And for those without learning difficulties, it can enhance abilities and improve those that are lagging.

On a body level, having your left and right brain integrated is the difference between having to look at your left land, making an L, to know it's your left. Now you can just 'know' intrinsically where your left is.

This makes an enormous difference to navigation for example. That little mistake can cost you your driving test. This is also the case for reversing or reverse parking. Looking over one shoulder and trying to manoeuvre a vehicle is very difficult without the spatial awareness you have when both left and right are well integrated. I have worked with many people who are so frustrated by the fact they cannot pass their driving test. You have no independence, and you feel like a second-class citizen. Especially where I live, as it's so rural – there is no public transport to compensate.

Emotionally, the left-right brain connections, if not balanced, can leave you feeling very unbalanced! The left brain, traditionally seen as the rational brain, balances out the free fall emotions that the right brain must process. Without this balance, we can find ourselves in an emotional loop we cannot get out of, as the left brain can't come in and rationalise for us.

Equally, if we are too left brained, we may feel little emotion, and instead, try to problem solve or make lists to try and understand what we are feeling. If we are this way with friends when they are sharing their troubles with us, they may feel unheard and misunderstood. In the long run, our friends may find us cold and disconnected, even thinking of us as being unemphatic.

Or we may experience social anxiety, as we realise we are not quite connecting with others in 'the proper way'. We may always have a 'slightly on the outside' feeling we carry even when amongst friends.

We may be liable to procrastinate with certain tasks as we find them too hard to do, and therefore, we can become rather set in the way we do things, once we have worked them out. This may lead to difficulties in adapting to others in our lives when we have closer relationships.

When our being is balanced, we are more able to stay in a state of high vibration. It is more difficult for the outside world to trigger us into a reaction or even trauma. We know our true selves so well that, even if we are temporarily taken off kilter, we know exactly how to return to ourselves. This confidence in knowing who we are will feed into an understanding of our place in the world, our role in this life and our part to play in the cosmos. We will hold strongly to our beliefs, but be open to listening to others' beliefs, not being unbalanced in our responses. Our inner knowing will be stronger, and this will help us navigate and make decisions in life with ease. We know what we want, and we know how to manifest it.

What is interesting about the ATNR on this topic, is that the dysfunction it causes in our sensory system could put us straight back into survival mode when the sensory system triggers us. Then we have to regulate either the FPR or the Moro or both, all over again. It's a little bit of a negative cycle. However, if we have worked extensively with the FPR and Moro, we will already have strategies in place to regulate ourselves. This really is the reason why we make sure we are ready, having worked on the Survival Reflexes before we do the 'higher' Reflexes.

My lack of time awareness was legendary amongst my students. It was like a lack of spatial awareness but with time. I always underestimated how much time it takes to get somewhere, or how much time it would take to leave a building, get to my car, not to mention any anomalies like tractors (I live rurally, so read traffic if you are city based!) It was always a running joke in my family, and I always put it down to the fact that I'm Peruvian and in Peru they have something called 'English time' and 'Peruvian time'. If you were invited to a party, it was normally Peruvian time (2 hours after stated time) and if it was a flight you had to catch, English time (i.e. be there when stated). So, I believed, I just ran on Peruvian time! It was well into my own Reflex Yoga journey before I realised a couple of things.

1. I was no longer late for anything.
2. I had a clear picture in my head of the coming week's appointments/classes/activities.
3. I was calculating time to get to places differently.
4. I was more aware of the passing of time.

Suddenly, I had become 'English!' Of course, this wasn't the case – I was always English, but I found that I was better 'connected' to time.

More difficult to pinpoint than my ability to measure time, I have also seen an improvement in organisational skills. I can remember where I put things and what I went upstairs to get, once I reach the top of the stairs! I now remember what my week looked like, including the odd appointments that aren't routine. I never leave any of my belongings behind anymore. I used to be the one who only realised they had left their coat behind when I walked out the door and realised I was cold!

Emotionally, I am also far more balanced. I was the sort of person that when upset, I would lose myself in the emotions, often shutting myself off under the duvet to really swim in the ocean of feelings. There's nothing wrong with that unless it lasts weeks and then makes it impossible for projects, work and family to thrive. I was so blown off track, I could even forget for months at a time my real mission in life. These days, I still feel all the feelings. However, there is another part of me which allows me to watch with much better equanimity, know that these feelings will pass as all things change, and be able to pick my life up much quicker. More importantly, I can differentiate between what feelings need to affect me and which belong to others. I can ascertain when someone is not angry at me, they are just angry in themselves – then I need not respond.

Spiritually integrating the ATNR has helped me to achieve an almost constant level of connection to my inner being. I know this is difficult to quantify for most of us, it certainly was for me. "What is an inner being?" I would always ask myself when I heard this phrase – it didn't make sense to me. Now I know it is a constant sense of inner knowing, an access to my deeper wisdom that I used to only be able to access in deeper meditation. My intuition, as some would call it, is spot on. When my body has a feeling, I can tune into it and make sense of what it is telling me. I can read a person, for example, much more easily. Are they hostile towards me, or in a negative space in themselves? With this deeper sense, I can stand in forgiveness and gratitude more constantly, understanding that human experience is not easy for any of us.

The ATNR exists to assist us with the birthing process by slowing down limb movements so that the baby can 'corkscrew' down the birth canal. In the womb, it provides stimulation to the muscle tone and the vestibular (balance) centres. You can see this in babies when the infant turns their head and the shoulder and arm stretch straight whereas the other arm is bent (this is why it is sometimes referred to as the 'Fencing Reflex') The movement is reversed when the head turns in the opposite direction, making it homolateral.

The left and right brain hemispheres are stimulated separately by movement. This Reflex helps the myelination of the corpus callosum. The corpus callosum oversees sending information between the two hemispheres. If this exchange of information is slow, we will have hemispheric preference being more right or left brained.

As this Reflex becomes integrated and more fine-tuned, it will help to integrate eye movements. We need to be able to coordinate both eyes to have binocular vision. Eye coordination is more important than you would first imagine. It has a significant effect on the maturation of the developmental arc and a major influence on complex development like speech and language.

The ATNR is also a Postural Reflex as it engages the muscles of the head, neck and trunk. It has a huge influence on a person's physical make up and coordination as it affects bilateral and cross-lateral coordination. As humans, we need to know our centre, our midline, so that we have healthy proprioception, movement control, spatial awareness and movement planning. The midline acts as a point of reference when planning our movement. And when it is well integrated, our movements become intuitive and flow easily. Being able to cross the midline (cross-lateral work) is important for sports but also for using cutlery, for example. In school children, the inability to participate well in sports can be a contributor towards feelings of isolation and inadequacy. In adults, we see a lot of 'crook' neck when this Reflex is retained and in more severe cases, migraines.

In our sensory system, the ATNR teaches the brain to hear with both ears. It acts as an interpreter of sounds and images and allows for the conversion and understanding of what you are seeing and hearing. Conversion means to be able to converge skills from one information processor to another. For example, auditory instruction into action or visual information in to written information.

When this Reflex is retained, we will likely be a forceps baby or a baby that never rolled or crawled. As we grow older, we may find one side of the body significantly more dominant than the other. We may clap using one hand more than the other, for example. We may lean towards one side and walk into the person we are talking to as we stride down the street. You may find that your balance is affected when you turn your head and so you cannot ride a bicycle, or you drop things when you turn your head.

In writing by hand, you may experience difficulties in holding the pen, gripping it too hard and pressing down too much. Writing the number 8 may be hard and there may be challenges when expressing ideas or creative writing. If the ATNR is retained, there will be significant reading challenges and as such it is the most present Reflex in people with dyslexia. Working with this Reflex will help a great deal in improving reading and learning.

When this Reflex is retained, we are distracted and easily overwhelmed, flitting from one task to another, never completing any. We find it hard to follow instructions and so find it tiresome to do so. In teens we may see body disassociation and body dysmorphia particularly in girls but not exclusively.

Working with this Reflex will see improvements to all of the above. You will experience better coordination and muscle strength, better visual and auditory processing skills and have more energy as a result. You may surprise yourself and be more eager to read, study or complete creative tasks as your ability to focus improves.

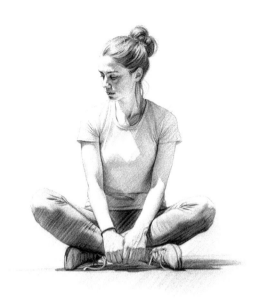

INTEGRATING THE ATNR

Before you begin your practice, do a couple of these exercises to ascertain how well your left and right brain work together.

Draw a large figure of 8 on the floor using chalk or marking the centre of the 8 with a pillow and the circles of the 8 with another two pillows. Now you can start walking the 8. Can you follow the figure without stopping? Do you hesitate when crossing the middle? After a while do you forget where you are and where to go next?

Grab a bean bag or a ball and pass it from one hand to another in front of you. Now try to pass it from one hand to another behind your back. See if you can then do one pass in front, one pass behind. Do you find it difficult? Are you getting stressed trying to remember whether it is time to pass at the front or back?

Head Turns

Lie down and place an object, say a ball on either side of your head. Now turn your head to look at one of the balls and then slowly rotate your head to look at the other ball. Once you have done this once or twice see if you can bring a slow rhythm into the movement. Make sure you are moving your eyes from ball to ball as the head turns.

Cross-lateral Crawl (Front and Back)

Either lying down or standing up bring your hand to an opposite knee. Repeat with the other hand to the other knee. Now begin to repeat rhythmically opposite hand to opposite knee, opposite hand to opposite knee until you feel like you can't do anymore or 2 minutes, whichever is the soonest.

When you have mastered this, try standing up, and this time crossing the hand to the opposite foot, behind you. Opposite hand to opposite foot, opposite hand to opposite foot, in rhythm. This is considerably trickier as you cannot see what you are doing. However, keep trying until it comes to you.

Eye Exercises

Place an object like a ball or a scarf in front of your eyes. Centre it so that both eyes are looking at it evenly. Make sure the distance is OK too. Now begin to move the ball up then down, up then down a few times. Side to side, side to side a few times. Now try up down, side to side. See how it feels. If you are feeling a little taxed, stop.

When you can do the above with ease add following the ball vertically and then in a circle and finally near to far. Again, all in rhythm and slowly!

The Lizard

Lie on your back with your body straight and turn your head to the right. Then as you stroke the right foot up your left leg, lift the same arm (the right) towards your head. Look at your arm. Now slowly stroke your foot down the leg and bring the other leg up, changing your arms around and turning your head to look the other way. Keep swapping sides a few times.

When you feel confident doing it lying on your back, try it on your front. Again, as it's harder to see your limbs, this is not as easy.

Cobra Integration

Lie on your front and bring your hands beneath your shoulders. Gently push up until you have most of your chest off the floor. Now look towards your left, notice what is happening in your right elbow. Do the same as you look towards your right, feel the left elbow become a little bit weaker. Try not to compensate for this weakness. Just know that it is there.

OTHER YOGIC EXERCISES FOR INTEGRATING THE FPR

Alternate Nostril Breathing

Sitting comfortably, bring your thumb to cover your right nostril and breathe in through your left nostril.
Now swap sides and place your finger over the left nostril, breathe out through this nostril and then breathe in again.
Swap around and cover your right nostril again, breathe out and then in again. Keep swapping between thumb and finger, covering each nostril in turn and breathing out then in. Keep it

rhythmic but don't worry too much about counting. Try it for one or two minutes.

Butterfly Tapping

In a seated or standing position, cross your arms over your heart, bringing the flats of your palms against your breastbone. Begin to tap the breastbone, first with one hand, and then the other in a rhythmic manner. Tap one side then tap the other, one side and then the other. Once the rhythm is established you could add, "I am calm," "I am peace," "I am joy," as you tap. Now cross your arms the other way and start again.

Relaxation

Start your relaxation with lip stroking (see Feet Hands Face) but this time you are also turning your head from one side to the other. Stroke your cheek from ear to chin, as you turn your head towards your shoulder.

Stop stroking your chin but continue to turn your head towards your shoulder until it is all the way around.

Repeat on the other side.

Once you have done this a few times, move the head back to the centre and begin to follow your breathing. As you begin to relax and you feel you are drifting away, have a final idea of the lip stroking you did – see if it will help you to relax even further.

AFFIRMATIONS:

"My body is relaxed."
"I feel my softness."
"I am balanced and ready to learn."

"I turn towards love and light."

OTHER ACTIVITIES FOR INTEGRATING ATNR:

- Canoeing
- Basketball
- Tennis
- Rounders (Baseball)

WHAT TO DO IF YOUR ATNR REFLEX IS OVERSTIMULATED

Signs that you may have overdone it in the ATNR include feeling tension in your neck, jaw clenching, feeling tired or feeling like giving up. If you ignore these signs, you may have red ears, feel nauseous or dizzy and perhaps unsteady on your feet.

If this occurs, try some of these exercises to help the nervous system calm down:

Lie down and make your neck comfortable. Place an eye pillow over your eyes and relax by feeling into your Feet Hands and Face.

Tap with tiny little taps, using both hands around the eyes until you feel them relax.

Cradle your head in your hands and press into the points that are a bit sore, just above each eyebrow. Feel your eyes relax.

CASE STUDY

B is a 14-year-old girl who I have worked with over the past three years, who has dyslexia and dyspraxia. Once she started her GCSE year, the added stress created chaos in her nervous system, making it harder to keep the connectivity that she already had in play.

As a teenager, there was also the added fact that her brain was in a process of pruning and changing, and her amygdala was more active. Anxiety levels had risen dramatically due to this, but also because now there was pressure to perform, to do well and pass tests. The stress of getting good grades and being seen to do well, was taking its toll.

Of course, my first port of call was to relax her system, make it feel safe, so that we could then work on the left-right brain connections as well as the other Reflexes. It's a good job we had time before the real pressure started, as it took us the best part of a year to work up from the Survival Reflexes, the Landau and STNR and finally to the ATNR. I have many pleasant memories of rolling around on the floor, learning how to roll 'properly'.

What was most interesting to me, is that finally the schoolwork was beginning to make sense, particularly in maths. We had gone from a place where it was flying over her head and she couldn't keep up, to a place where, with attention and effort, she could do the work. The school were now happy to put her forward for the examinations and three years after we started, she took her exams with pride.

ATNR IN YOGA PRACTICE

The ATNR Reflex is an important Reflex for many of us. From time to time, we all have problems with our necks and most of us have experienced a stiff neck at least once in our lives. Crook neck is a common complaint in the general population. You will be happy to know that you can help yourself with this on a physical level as well as everything else.

It is also important to point out to you that we will be working on right left-brain integration, and that there may be moments when there is 'interference' or an inability to coordinate both sides of the body and brain. I have found that having some forewarning makes it a less confusing experience, as we are expecting it at some time during our sessions. It is always good to point out the benefits of working through these moments of lack of coordination as it encourages us to keep trying, even if we are finding it hard.

No doubt there will be a lot of work for you to do, to coordinate your left-right movement, so be attentive and observant if you are struggling, or if you are unable to do the movements in a coordinated way. If you become overwhelmed, do some of the exercises above to help.

METHOD 1 – MOVEMENT LEFT TO RIGHT, IN ASANA

Once you have completed some of the integration exercises, it is good to keep the movement going with some asanas that are like the integration exercises. And to use them to help cement the patterns made in integration.

For example, in Seated Twist Pose:

As you sit on the floor in a cross-legged position, bring your opposite hand onto your opposite knee and at the same time look over your shoulder. Now close your eyes so they don't strain and imagine you are looking even further over your shoulder. Notice how this helps to get you a little bit further. Now repeat on the other side.

Other poses that may work well with this method include:

Lying Twists

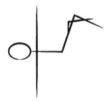

Cobra (look left to right while in Cobra)

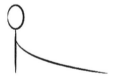

Bridge (look left to right)

Tree Pose

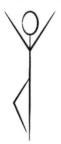

METHOD 2 – FEELING THE SHOULDER-NECK CONNECTION

When integrating this Reflex, particularly when doing the Cobra Integration above, you can feel how the hands, arms, shoulders, neck and eyes are interconnected. In this method, we pay special attention to the shoulders and neck connection and use this awareness to help relax and release any tension in the shoulders.

I have found that it is important to do a before and after Cobra Integration Exercise, so you can really feel the difference in how you are able to relax the shoulders. After all the integration exercises that you have chosen to do have been done, go back to the Cobra Integration and do it again, so you can feel the isolation and relief in the shoulders. Then use this awareness to remind yourself to stretch in the asanas with relaxed shoulders.

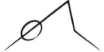

For example, in Downward Dog:

On all fours, come into Downward Dog, settle your shoulders

into the relaxed feeling they had at integration. Then move your head from side to side and see if you can feel the isolation felt earlier whilst in this pose. You can also visualise in your head doing the Cobra Integration Exercise again. Enquire as to what difference this makes to the pose.

Other yoga poses where this may also be achieved are:

Standing Forward Bend

Puppy Pose

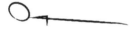

Chair Pose

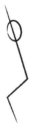

Plank Pose

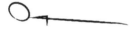

METHOD 3 – FEELING THE NECK-EYE CONNECTION

This method is very similar to the above, only now we use the eyes to help the neck stretch further and so also allow the shoulders to relax more. As this method uses the eyes and is much more powerful, I'd recommend you use this method after you have had a few experiences with the ATNR already, so that your system is more resilient, and you do not become too tired. Once you have moved into a yoga pose, close your eyes and direct your eyes either to the left or right whilst they are in asana. Feel the difference this makes to the stretch; and by bringing your attention fully to it, you can integrate this Reflex better.

For example, Seated Knot Twist:

Sitting on the floor, bend one leg under the other and bring the other leg over that leg's knee. Bringing the opposite hand toward the opposite knee. There are various ways to hold that leg – either with the hand or with the middle of the arm, or by bringing the whole arm over the knee, depending on your flexibility.

Turn your head to look over the shoulder as far as you can, and then close your eyes and move the eyes to the right or left depending on which side you are working. Acknowledge any difference you feel in your shoulders as they release.

Other yoga poses that work well with this are:

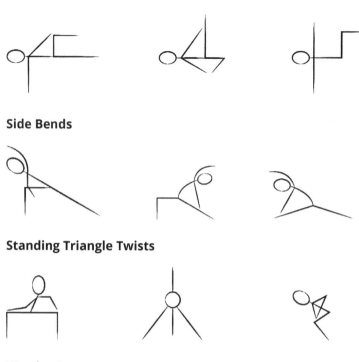

Side Bends

Standing Triangle Twists

Warrior Poses

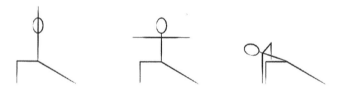

Imagine that the top of your head is a circle and in it is surrounded by a box. Tilt your head back towards one of the corners of the box. Now centre the head. Tilt it back towards the other corner of the box. Centre the head. Now tilt the head forward towards the front corner of the box. Centre. Tilt the head towards the other front corner. Centre.

Now turn your chin towards one shoulder and tilt your head towards the back corner of the box. Centre. turn your chin toward the other shoulder tilt back to the other corner. Centre. Turn your chin toward the other shoulder tilt to a forward corner. Centre. Turn your chin towards the other shoulder and tilt to the other forward corner. Centre.

Now take in what you can feel in the neck, base of the skull, jaw and throat. What does this new neurological pattern feel like for you. See if you can remember it and use it as you do some stretching for the neck and spine.

CONCLUSION

Although very subtle, there are distinct sensations in the body, once this Reflex is better integrated. We are barely aware of them, but we are better coordinated and able to navigate our bodies through space. This also gives us confidence in our body's ability to complete complex tasks, which makes us feel competent. We become more aware of our abilities and can harness them to accomplish difficult tasks, knowing that we may need time to 'think things through' and 'work it out.' There is no longer an emotional response to having to do difficult things, as we know we can give it a go and ask for help if necessary.

Naturally we become better organised, sometimes without even noticing; and so life flows easily, giving us a sense of things being as they should be. We no longer worry if something doesn't turn out as it should, knowing that if it is important enough, we can try again or put what is wrong right. These measured responses are signs of good left-right brain balance, and they permeate through all our decision making, organising and what of life. We are 'level-headed' and able to use all our abilities to succeed in life.

We may find we do tasks that before felt out of our reach with ease, only realising later that we have accomplished something we never thought we could. We can reverse the car a mile down a single-track lane, or we pass our driving test at last. Our nervous system will not fly into fight/flight/freeze/fawn mode so easily, as we keep ourselves balanced and steady through the ups and downs of life.

RAGGED CIRCLES

I wish my mind would stop running ragged circles
Around the jagged edges of my heart.
Then maybe the craggy corners will
Smooth themselves out at last.

Veronika Peña de la Jara

CHAPTER 8

The Landau Reflex

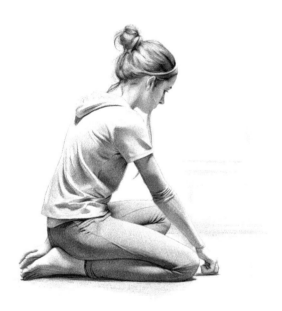

Being stuck in the Landau brings a lot of rigidity and uncomfortableness. The spine is in a perpetual action of extension and the muscles around it must be tight and tense to support this unconscious action.

The same is the case for the emotional and spiritual body. One must feel constantly working so hard to reach for what one wants, and striving is a constant companion. It is difficult to 'just be'. We often feel alone, as we are the only ones who 'can do it right' – frustration settling in easily with ourselves and others. Eventually we may burn out from trying so hard to achieve something, anything. The middle child in a family of three siblings will be either a fighter for their rights or will surrender completely. Mostly I see them surrender. However occasionally I do see a child who is on fire! Demanding the attention they so rightfully need.

On the other side, if we have not even emerged this Reflex, we may find that we are listless, and never reach for anything. There is little ambition or drive, and life feels like a chore, something just to get through, and again it is a lonely place to be. There is little point to anything it seems, so why bother. Our attitude to life is flat and we are often bored, switched off to the opportunities and possibilities right in front of us.

I often think of the middle child of three in a family with this Reflex, having to give in on attention to the baby and having a dominant older sibling who is used to getting attention, the one in the middle 'gives' up and takes whatever comes their way, if it ever does. The general demeanour is to surrender to the demands of those around her as it is just easier.

When we have managed to either release the strong hold of this Reflex or to introduce its pattern into the body, many things change. We can begin to reach for what we need at any given moment and actualise our dreams without the need to fight for it. We just know we deserve to. We can push through the obstacles in our way without bulldozing those around us. And we can measure our stamina so that we don't wear ourselves out. There will be a more balanced approach to achieving our aims and desires which includes considering others and their help and support. We don't need to do everything alone and life becomes a journey, not a destination.

Spiritually, we can understand that we are part of the whole –

nothing is demanded of us, we can just be who we are. Our sense of who that is, is becoming more defined as we reach for the things that make us feel good, put us on the vibration of happiness and joy, knowing we deserve it just because. No reasons are needed. We are a child of the Universe, here to achieve something good because we are good, we carry the Divine light within, and we mean to shine it bright into the world.

The Landau, like the Spinal Galant is a transitional Reflex, which comes online initially to gain muscle tone in the neck and back. When you see a baby engaging these muscles for the first time, they are in Landau Reflex. Without this Reflex we will have low muscle tone in the neck making the next Reflex, the TLR, difficult to integrate. In the worst cases, it can lead to an inability to lift the head or a hunched back therefore, it is important for overall postural stability and then for the ability for the baby to extend its hands and arms and reach out and grab something they have seen that they want to explore. First, they learn to lift their head and then the chest, freeing the arms to reach. Being able to lift the head also begins to integrate near vision and 3D vision, as the eyes can now see what is in front of them.

You may see the lack of integration physically in this Reflex, particularly when learning to swim, for example. The legs extend when head is bent backwards and so you tire easily. The upper or lower body feels weak and either one or the other is overly tense. Without this reflex properly integrated, we may feel clumsy, walking into things and have tense legs which are prone to extend backwards.

Within the nervous system, we are learning to establish a clear distinction between the upper and lower body, and it is key for connecting the neocortex to the prefrontal cortex, giving us better attention, concentration and memory. If this Reflex is retained, we may experience short term memory loss. This Reflex is also enabling our vestibular, proprioception and vision senses to process and organise the difference between up and down.

My personal experience of this Reflex has been very noticeable. I had always been someone who started something and never quite managed to finish it. I would get as far as 90% there, yet that last bit would never quite happen. Sometimes to the point that I just decided it was finished at 90%, when I knew it was not! Even tasks that I knew would benefit me or would give me joy would never quite make it to the end.

It wasn't until recently that I realised that I was completing tasks. I hadn't even noticed. I realised that the blocks I usually had were because there was a part of the task, I found difficult. I felt I couldn't do it myself and I was not reaching out for help. I have learnt to know my limitations and to reach out to experts to help me finish off my work.

A great example of this was my website. A few years ago, I had taken a 'Build Your Own Website' course which had taught me how to set up a basic website. What it didn't do, however, was teach me how to fine tune it, and I could tell it wasn't quite up to scratch when I had done all I could do. I'm not sure, maybe there were modules I didn't finish... Instead of leaving it as it was, I reached out and paid for someone to come along and tweak it for me until I was happy. It looks amazing!

Reaching out for help has spread in my life – from simple things like asking my family to do more around the house, to deeper inner work with a therapist – I have begun to have a sense that I don't have to do it all alone. I am no longer hyper-independent. What is interesting, however, is that I feel more capable in myself at the same time, so my need to reach out is more practical than emotional and less frequent. Before it was the other way around, I'd move hell or high water to achieve something in the practical realm but was very co-dependent, particularly for work-related activities. I wouldn't run yoga days without someone else helping me and the thought of running women's groups was out of the question. Nowadays, I do both alone. I do however ask for help if I need it!

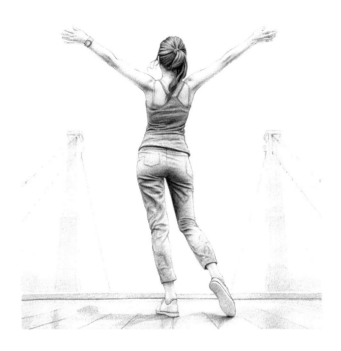

MOVEMENTS TO INTEGRATE THE LANDAU

Before you begin, you may well want to find out if this Reflex is affecting you. And if so, how much? There is an easy way to do this. Lie down on the floor with your tummy on the ground, your arms by your sides. Now, lift your head and chest at the same time a few times. Is there a lot of difficulty lifting your head and chest? Do your legs lift slightly when your head is up? Is there tension in your legs? Are you tightening your buttocks as you lift? How does your neck feel? Is it tense? Does the neck shake or clench? Is there pain and if so, where?

Please feel free to visit **www.the-empowered-feminine.co.uk** for a Landau-based yoga practice example. At the end of this book, there are details of how to access the videos that accompany this book.

www.the-empowered-feminine.co.uk

Isometric Head

Lying on your back place a hand on your forehead and apply some pressure there as you try and lift the head off the ground, then let go. Repeat three times. Notice how your neck and upper back feel after this.

Roll over onto your front and place a hand on the back of the head and push into the floor, resisting with your head, recreating the same amount of pressure as before. Let go and repeat three times. Again, have a moment to feel into how your neck and upper back respond to this.

Superman

Lie on your front with your arms stretched out in front of you and raise you head and chest, trying to relax your legs (think FPR) as you lift. Keep the arms on the ground for now.

Take a few breaths focusing on the out-breath, and then lift your arms up above the head, lifting the arms head and chest for a few more breaths.

As you come down to rest, focus on what is happening in your body. Where can you feel tension releasing?

Longitudinal Rock

Lie on your front with your hands beneath your shoulders. Let your toes curl under and lift your head in line with the back, not too high.

Begin to use your hands and feet to gently rock yourself backwards and forwards in a rhythmic manner. When you have a gentle rhythm going, begin to switch between using your hands to power the movement (letting the legs relax) and then relaxing the hands and letting the feet power the movements. When your feet are tired, use both hands and feet again for a while and repeat the cycle: using hands, feet and both in turn. Keep it up for a minute or two, no more.

When you have finished, remember to relax a moment and feel the effects on your body.

WHAT TO DO IF YOU FEEL YOU ARE LANDAU TRIGGERED

If you feel a sharp back, chest or neck pain, bring your body into a Knee to Chest Pose and take some deep breaths. Allow your attention to come back to your Feet Hands and Face as you breathe deeply. If you feel that you are a bit panicky, add to the attention of Feet Hands and Face, a visual focal point which you can gently focus on. You can also apply pressure to the nape of the neck or use a heavy bean bag.

As always if you feel triggered, stop the practice for now and work on the Survival Reflexes, the Feet Hands and Face and the STNR, until you are ready to try again.

OTHER EXERCISES FOR INTEGRATING THE LANDAU

RAISING AWARENESS WITH LANDAU

Find a way to sit comfortably, but without leaning back on anything. Try to have your spine free. As you close your eyes, begin to be aware of your breathing, just noticing it as it comes in and out. Now begin to take your awareness to your spine and notice that as you breathe in, very subtly, your spine reaches upwards and as you breathe out, again almost unnoticeably, it comes back into a C position.

If at first you can't feel the reach of the spine, keep your attention mostly on the outbreath. Feeling the slight collapse of the spine in C position is often easier to feel. Now once again observe the in-breath and see if you can feel the spine reaching, moving gently into an S shape.

AFFIRMATIONS

"I am connected to my body."
"I am connected to my inner being."
"I can achieve whatever I set out to achieve."
"Everything is always working out for me."
"I deserve to receive my deepest desires."

OTHER ACTIVITIES GOOD FOR LANDAU:

- Climbing
- Monkey bars
- Pull ups

- Swimming (Front Crawl particularly)
- Silks and hoop work

INTEGRATED LANDAU IN YOGA PRACTICE

When working with the Landau, we have learnt that the main physical effect is learning to differentiate the upper from the lower body, especially when reaching, which is a cue that is given a lot in yoga practice. It is therefore important to make sure that you start any asana with raised awareness of grounding the feet and relaxing the legs and back (see FPR). Then it will be possible to direct the upper body to lift and move in a healthier way. In this Reflex, we really want to learn how to reach without tensing the lower back and legs, so keep remembering how the legs feel in FPR when you reach up with your arms or spine.

It is also very possible that you are unconsciously holding your lower and upper body together and this work can really help to highlight this for us. When we become aware of this unconscious holding pattern, it is possible to release it much more effectively, not just when practicing yoga, but in daily life. We can also use this Reflex to help manage upper and lower body movement. Especially if we bring the Spinal Galant work into it. Working these two Reflexes together can really work wonders. You could do a few Spinal Galant exercises first and then feel into whether the lower two hotplates are sinking down towards the earth as the top two move upwards.

METHOD 1 – SINKING THE BACK AND BREATHING UP THE BODY

Healthy moving when practicing asanas, is about using your body in a way that is efficient as well as comfortable. Avoiding using too many muscles that are not necessarily needed in movement. So, after some Landau Integration moves like the ones above, we are best placed to really feel the body moving in a new, more relaxed way. You can ask yourself to really feel the downward feeling of the lower body, and breathe into the chest and feel the upward motion of the lungs being full.

For example, in Dynamic Dandasana:

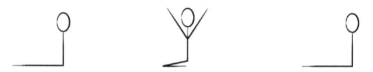

While in sitting position, really feel the sitting bones let go into the earth and relax the legs as much as possible. To begin with, just breathe in this position and feel the breath lift the upper body away from the floor, whilst leaving the lower body where it is.

Once you have processed this, you can begin to use movements of the arms as you breathe. Opening the arms out as you breathe in, and forward folding as you breathe out. This is a dynamic move and so is harder than the static breathing, but it can easily highlight if there is a holding pattern going on as you move.

Other poses that work well with this method are:

Yogic Breath

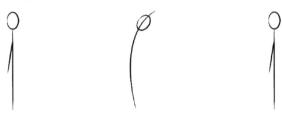

Hero Pose

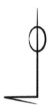

METHOD 2 – ANCHORING DOWN THROUGH THE PELVIS

With this method, we are being more specific about where our attention is going. We need to bring more awareness during our integration stage to the downward release of the pelvis itself. So, make sure you choose integration exercises that give this feedback – like the Locust.

Concentrate on the heavy feeling in the pelvis (better done on the floor) – where the pelvis sits on the ground – and the downward pull of the sitting bones. Make sure that the tail is fanning out and the belly is soft, as this will benefit most women and is the correct position for a woman's pelvis.

Having embodied the pelvis and really felt into it, it's position and weight, it is time to begin to move into asana.

For example, in Staff Pose:

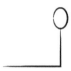

Sit down with your legs stretched out in front of you. If you are uncomfortably leaning backwards, bend your legs slightly and if it still feels difficult, then perhaps a bolster beneath your knees will help. What is important is to be able to relax whilst the spine is straight.

Lean slightly forward and fan out your tail behind you and return to sitting upright. See if this feels any more comfortable and really feel into where the sitting bones are and where the pelvis sits. If you want, after this you can move this into a Forward Fold position now.

Other asanas where this method is useful are:

All sitting poses, forward bends and twists

In standing poses, feel the pelvis above the legs like a bowl on a stand

Fish Pose

Locust Pose

Childs Pose

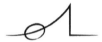

Puppy Pose

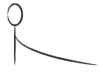

METHOD 3 – COMPARING NOT SEPARATING, TO RELEASING AND SEPARATING

In this method, we are deliberately moving the body in two ways to compare them to each other and further integrate the Reflex within our movement. The idea is to compare how one movement feels with a holding pattern between upper and lower body and then to do the same asana with these separated. For this method, it can also be useful to remind ourselves of the four hotplates and the 3D movement patterns we worked with in the Spinal Galant.

For example, in the Cobra Pose:

Lie on your front and tighten your buttocks, as you push up through the hands to do the Cobra Pose. Feel how the tightness is in the body and the breath. When this is done, do some of the integration exercises like the Locust or the Longitude Rock. Then you can repeat the asana and feel the difference.

Other poses that work well with this method are:

Standing Back Bend

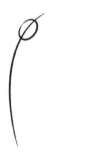

Reverse Plank Pose

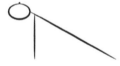

Bridge Pose

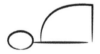

Hands Free Cobra

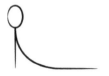

CONCLUSION

To have the drive to achieve one's dream and see them through thick and thin, you need to be able to reach for the stars. As they say, reach for the stars and see how far you will go! Dreaming big and being confident that you can get there, is the result of a well-integrated Landau. Taking the steps to reach your goals will seem easy when this Reflex is in full flow. You will be able to seek help when you get stuck and when things aren't easy, you will not give up. You will find a way around the obstacle, whether it is practical, mental or spiritual.

You will find that as you are active in moving forward in your life, to achieve your goals, you will also be more relaxed in getting there. There will be an underlying understanding that, to be relaxed, helps. It means you are better connected internally to your sense of self, and delays will just appear to be part of the journey. You will no longer be frustrated or angry when things go wrong. You won't blame others, instead you will reach for the moral support you need, regroup, relax and keep on moving forward. As you relax more, your confidence will grow. You begin to feel that you know you will reach your goal. Nothing can stop you.

Your body will be so grateful that you no longer push it to its limit and tire yourself out. Gone is the tension in your lower back and legs and the energy released here will help keep you energised, as your whole body now has access to the energy that the tension took up. You will walk through the world, relaxed, upright and moving forward in life.

SOVEREIGN MOTHER

I am becoming something new,
In this changing paradigm of life.
Some call it single motherhood,
I prefer Sovereign Mother.

I am Sovereign Mother to myself first,
As I stand in Harmony and Love.
Not being pushed in all directions by others,
Only in stability I command.

I am becoming, becoming, becoming,
Every moment of every day.
Every cell rearranging itself
In a healthier way.

I am Queen of my world and
In this next stage of my life,
I will be the mother of women and men,
Who will soon be Sovereign too.

I am a Sovereign Mother,
I am becoming something new.
I am peace, harmony and love,
Who will birth something true.

Veronika Peña de la Jara

CHAPTER 9

Tonic Labyrinthic Neck Reflex

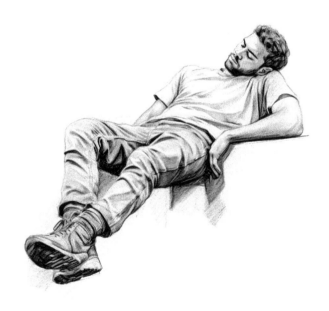

This is the one Reflex I do not regularly cover in my yoga classes, as it sits on top of all the others. There is so much work to do before we can fully integrate the TLR. Every so often, I venture to do a session in the TLR, and it is always so well received. The main reason is the effect it has on releasing neck tension. Those with neck pain of any kind always request this Reflex when given a choice.

Physically, when we are using the TLR to release the neck we can expect to see changes in posture. The position we hold our neck in will have an effect all the way down to the shoulder, spine and pelvis alignment. The head is heavy! If it is not sitting comfortably where it should be on top of the neck, then we will have different parts of our body compensating for us. Reasons for having a tilt in the head position may vary.

For me, it was that I have one stronger eye than the other, so when I need bifocal viewing, I turn my head slightly to the side. You could also have one ear hearing better than the other, which could cause this slight turn of the head. If you have been doing this sort of head turning all your life, it will seem normal to have the head slightly tilted or turned towards one side and as the inner ear, tells the rest of your body where your head is in space, changing this can be tricky and long winded. However, doing so will release a lot of tension in the neck and shoulders, as they will have had to work extra to keep the head in what is in effect an unnatural position.

Having independent movement of the head from the body feels so freeing. It is almost as if the head is floating above the body and feels so much less work to carry. The shoulders can relax more, and the head feels more stable, sitting in its correct position. The eyes take less effort to look around you, avoiding eye strain and having better eye to body coordination which makes our sensory system calmer.

Emotionally, we are not startled quite so easily. We have a better sense of what is around our head and so if something comes in from the outside suddenly (like a ball), we are more likely to see it and be able to move our head quickly to avoid it.

Because we are not easily startled, we are more confident in the world and able to face whatever comes our way. We are less likely to have a jerky reaction to what the world presents us, as we are calmer and more confident in ourselves. This also means that we are not thrown off our emotional stability that easily either. We can 'read' the room and the people in it, knowing what to expect. We have a better sense of what might come our way and so we are more emotionally prepared.

In traditional yoga, the position of the head was sometimes described as feeling like you had a thread which connected to the top of your head, which was suspended from above. I like this image as it helps us to understand the spiritual connection integrating the TLR can give us. If we have this golden thread connecting us to source, to spirit, to nature, dharma, call it what you will, we are able to trust the intuition we feel because we feel aligned with whatever greater power made us.

This brings more trust in ourselves, in the reasons we are here, potent energy in human form and so we can begin to feel gratitude and blessed that we have the awareness to be connected so. Our inner voice can be released, and we can open to say what is truly in our hearts.

For me personally this journey with the TLR began as I also worked with the Mouth-Jaw Reflex. The release I feel when working these two together is a sense of coming out of being strangled. Physically, this feeling comes around my throat but also into my upper back and under my armpits. When using the integration exercises, my whole body responds, and my level of awareness is raised. There is a sensation of drawing myself back into my body, as it has got distracted by my thoughts. I can now become present again. In this presence I also feel so connected that my inner self is nearby, helping me to navigate the world.

Alongside the physical work, as I have worked with this Reflex more and more, I cannot help but notice that my connection to spirit, to my intuition has improved. I know because I remember years ago trying to read the tarot cards for friends and being exhausted by it. These days I can connect like that without even thinking about it. This has paid off massively in my resent separation, where I have 'known' what shenanigans were going on behind my back. I was better prepared for what I suspected, and truly was going on. It did not stop this from affecting me emotionally – I still had to deal with that – but at least it was not so much a shock or surprise.

There are two parts to the TLR; forwards and backwards. The Reflex exists to help an infant adapt to the new world on land. Our first world is in water, and the way our body responds to water is so different. The gravitational conditions of land need to be assimilated and the TLR does this well. As the baby learns about this new world, it gains a new vestibular (balance centre) and proprioceptive sense. Muscles are formed in the body and limbs to react to the small movements of the head.

Slowly over the next 9 months, the baby will develop the ability to get into an upright, stable, balanced position without the front or the back of the body playing a greater role than the other.

If the Reflex is not well integrated, the body's ability to manage head movement either forward or backward will change the muscle tone. This confuses and stresses the balance centre and there can be difficulties in judging space, speed and distance. We have no sense of direction, left right or up down. Posture is affected, as the head feels too heavy to carry and we find ourselves leaning over the table with hunched back and weak neck muscles. We will then be using the rest of the body (legs folding under the chair or wrapped around the chair) to compensate. As the head is not in its correct position and it affects the rest of the body, you may see 'W' sitting, or a tendency to walk on the tip toes.

Having a poor sense of balance and coordination will bring

in a fear of heights and difficulties in walking on open steps (without risers). If you must look up or down while walking (say because the track is uneven) you find yourself unbalanced and this will lead to a lack of confidence in walking and running too. Activities involving head and leg coordination will be difficult. In swimming, for example, turning your head to breathe in front crawl and continuing kicking will be hard. Mostly you will stop kicking altogether.

If the TLR is not integrated well, the body's ability to manage head movement backward or forward, will change muscle tone involuntarily. This can confuse and stress the balance centre, and as a result, there can be greater difficulties in judging space, distance, depth and speed. We can have difficulties following directions and may experience hunched posture, weak neck muscles and problems with walking.

In worst cases, we may experience an eye squint or tic, have near to far eye convergence difficulties making reading difficult. With a low tone in the eye muscles, we may be cross-eyed too. An active TLR backwards can influence:

As the system is overworked and overloaded, there will be tiredness and, due to the body challenges and lack of dopamine, high anxiety levels. The body, and therefore the mind, will have delayed responses and be forgetful and disorganised. After a while, we will feel disillusioned in ourselves and therefore have low self-esteem. This will make us much more introverted and can, at its worst, make us uncommunicative. We may notice we have poor short-term memory.

Because we have so much happening in our body, as it tries to compensate for not really knowing what the head is doing, we don't have the space within to take time to understand how we are feeling. Despite the fact we have plenty of emotions, we are often out of touch with them, and do not understand our feelings very well. We may feel sensations, but we do not know what they mean. We cannot translate them.

TLR also has a connection to the amygdala gland in the centre of the brain, therefore it can trigger the fear and alert centres and dopamine exchange. Dopamine helps regulate movement, attention, learning, and emotional responses. It also enables us not only to see rewards but to take action to move toward them. Since dopamine contributes to feelings of pleasure and satisfaction, as part of the reward system, this neurotransmitter also plays a part in addiction. People with low dopamine may also be more prone to addiction. The presence of a certain kind of dopamine receptor is associated with sensation seeking, more commonly known as risk-taking.

As we have low levels of 'the happy hormone' dopamine and we do not have good access to the sensations we carry, we may not have a connection with our inner selves. Looking within may be depressing, as we just feel bad and we are cruising through life, trying our best to survive without any sense of what we are truly a part of. We may never even entertain the question: What is this life all about? Why am I here?

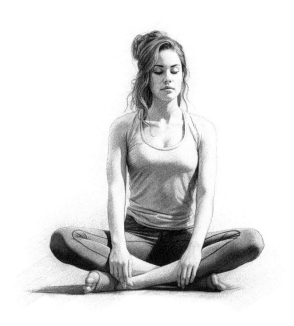

INTEGRATING THE TLR

As I have alluded to above, this Reflex is the last in a long line of work that may well take years to finish. If we imagine that the FPR is the roots of a tree, the Moro the heart, The STNR and ATNR the trunk, The Spinal Galant and Landau the reaching branches; then the TLR are the leaves and fruits of the tree. If the rest of the tree is not healthy then the benefits of the TLR cannot blossom. Therefore, it is important to work on the rest of the tree first and have those Reflexes well known in your body and nervous system before you attempt to do this Reflex intensely. There is no harm adding it to your lexicon of movement from time to time, we just need to know that it will be the last piece of the jigsaw to slot into place.

You can tell if you have a TLR (forward or backward) quite easily. Either ask someone, or film yourself standing upright and then simply look up and down. Can you move your head independently of your body or does your breastbone lift, and/ or your back arch, depending on which way you are looking?

PERSONAL PRACTICE

Please feel free to visit **https://the-empowered-feminine. co.uk/toolkit-free** for a hand-based yoga practice example. At the end of this book there are details as to how to access the videos that accompany this book.

www.the-empowered-feminine.co.uk

Begin by checking in with your body and your breath and afterwards have a moment to tune into how different you feel.

Perhaps answering some of these questions:

How did your neck feel as you were moving it in this new way? What aftereffects did you feel in the neck? Where there any aftereffects on other parts of your body? How much were you able to do before you realised your nervous system was over worked? Were you as resilient as you have been so far?

MOVEMENTS TO INTEGRATE THE TLR

Head Rolling

Bring yourself onto all fours and place your head on the floor. Start to roll it in, tucking the chin in towards the chest and then roll it back, trying to bring the chin and nose onto the floor.

Moving slowly, repeat as many times as feels comfortable. Try not to stretch your neck here, this is more about the movement pattern than stretching out the neck.

Isometric Head Holding and Pushing Against the Hand

Lie on the floor facing up and bring your hand to place it on your forehead. Now begin to push against it as if you were trying to lift your head off the floor but the hand was preventing you. Make sure the hand resists you lifting and then relax. Notice what muscles engage and relax as you repeat. Notice the relaxation that may also be present in the throat, jaw and palate.

Bring your right hand above your right ear. Now push your head into the hand, the hand resisting you so that you don't move. Again, feel what muscles are active and observe them as they relax.

Bring your left hand above the left year and again push your head into the hand, the left hand resisting you so that you don't move. Have a moment to feel the muscles you are using and how they feel after you have released them.

Now turn over and place your hands on the back of your head and repeat the same movement. Try to lift your head whilst the hands stop you. Feel the resistance and feel into the muscles that engage and how they relax when you let go.

Head Rocking Side to Side

Lie on your back. Gently move the head in a rhythmic manner side to side, as if you were saying 'no' but in very small movements. The movement side to side is as small as you can make it and the rhythm rapid. It is as if you are trying to 'unscrew' the head from the spine.

The Circle and the Square

Imagine that the top of your head is a circle and it is surrounded by a box. Tilt your head back towards one of the corners of the box. Now centre the head. Tilt it back towards the other corner of the box. Centre the head. Now tilt the head forward towards the front corner of the box. centre. Tilt the head towards the other front corner. Centre.

Now turn your chin towards one shoulder and tilt your head towards the back corner of the box. Centre. Turn your chin toward the other shoulder tilt back to the other corner. Centre. Turn your chin toward the other shoulder tilt to a forward corner. Centre. Turn your chin towards the other shoulder and tilt to the other forward corner. Centre.

Now take in what you can feel in the neck, base of the skull, jaw and throat. What does this new neurological pattern feel like for you? See if you can remember it and use it, as you do some stretching for the neck and spine.

Make sure as you are doing all these exercises that you are also paying attention to what is releasing in the throat, jaw and palate, as well as the release in the neck. These are more subtle sensations. However, they can also hold the head tightly in position if they are not released.

The Flagpole and the Rag

Pay attention to the position of your head and feel it directly above the spine – as if the spine was a flagpole and the head the rag that is about to polish it. Start moving the head in tiny circles at the top of the flagpole and gradually begin to grow the circles until you are polishing the whole of the top of the flagpole. Come back to the centre at the top of the flagpole and do the same in the other direction.

Come back to the centre again and this time, polish the flagpole in a side to side action, moving the chin towards one shoulder and back again. Do small movements and then carry this on as you tilt the head forwards as far as it will go, keeping it independent of spinal movement. Then come back to the centre and repeat this time with the head tilting backwards.

Bring your ear to your shoulder and now polish the flagpole over the top from ear to ear and back again. Do this a few times. Bring the head back to the centre and notice how it feels, how loose the head feels, how free.

Now imagine that you are trying to centre the head, but the flagpole is too greasy so it easily falls/slides off it, in whatever direction it feels like going. Keep doing this for as long as feels comfortable.

Once you are finished, you will know exactly where your head belongs.

WHAT TO DO IF YOU FEEL YOUR TLR IS TRIGGERED

As this Reflex affects the vestibular, be careful not to overdoing the TLR exercises, as this can lead to feelings of disorientation and dizziness. If you get any signs, stop immediately and rest. Do not move into another position, just keep yourself as still as possible, until the dizziness has passed and then stop working on this area until another time.

If dizziness is severe, then find a focal point to look at in the distance or nearer if there is no horizon to look at. Then orientate yourself to this point. Look at the point – where are you in relation to this? Ground yourself at the same time, feeling which parts of your body are touching the floor. Can you feel your feet? Where are your feet in relation to where you are looking at?

OTHER EXERCISES FOR INTEGRATING THE TLR

RAISING AWARENESS WITH THE TLR

This Reflex builds awareness of when and how we hold tension in the neck, throat, jaw and palate when doing asanas. Try to see what happens now when you listen to a gong or singing bowl placed in front of you, with the feeling of the sound moving forward into you. Now turn over and with a second gong or singing bowl feel the motion of the sound moving through the back of you. Is there a response in your neck, jaw or mouth? Which side elicited the response?

AFFIRMATIONS

"I hold myself up."
"I am balanced."
"I am connected to the great above."
"I am light."

OTHER ACTIVITIES TO DO TO HELP THE TLR INTEGRATE

- Swimming with the head in the water (all strokes)
- Climbing
- Tennis
- Hand ball games; dodge ball, netball, basketball

CASE STUDY

There is a lovely 93-year-old lady in one of my senior classes who has been doing yoga since the 1970s. For her age, she neither looks nor moves like she is over 90. Years of tuning into her body have kept her in good shape and everyone is always amazed when they are told her age. Many in the other 3 groups of senior yoga classes I hold, are in awe of her and are motivated by her health and vitality.

Despite all this work, however, when we lie down her head is slightly tilted towards the right, and she often requests that 'we do some neck work' as she suffers from tension and sometimes pain in her left shoulder. She now knows this is down to her head position. She does not remember why or if there was any trauma to her head or if she was born this way but this is the only part of her body now causing her trouble. At 93! Not bad.

Although we do not do the TLR that often in class, as she has been with me for years, she does know some of the integration exercises. Initially they did cause a little dizziness and slight nausea, yet now she assures me this is not the case. She tells me she practices the moves regularly, as it helps to relieve the pain in her shoulder. More and more often when we lie down to relax these days, her head is in its correct position.

YOGA WITH THE TLR INTEGRATED

Having practiced a few of the integration exercises above, try these poses to see how it feels, now your head is looser off the neck. Because the TLR is the Reflex at the end of our developmental arc, do try it in these simple poses first, so that you can continue to familiarise yourself with how it feels for your head to not be held on so tight before you try a full yoga session.

Downward Dog

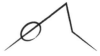

In Downward Dog, allow the head to be as loose as possible and gently look up and down trying to keep the neck as relaxed as possible so that it is independent of the spine.

Standing Forward Bend

As above, let your head move up and down but not so much that it moves the spine. You can also circle the head and move it side to side, to feel the difference as the head loosens off the spine and you can feel the head's weight.

Cobra

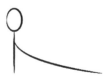

Lying down on your front, allow the lower back to relax into the ground and without lifting the head push the floor away from you and check that you are not tensing the neck as you do so. Then keeping the hands pushing, allow the upper back to lift, checking for any neck tension and trying to keep it relaxed. Tilt the head back gradually.

Standing Back Bend

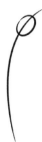

As you stand, bring your arms up ready to begin but check for any neck tension before you move. Bring the hips forward and the upper back backwards. Use your core, not your neck, to hold the position. Try and keep the head at the top of the 'flagpole' until the very end where you can tilt it back in a relaxed manner.

Half Headstand

As you put your head and arms into headstand position and bring the weight to bare on the base of the head, make sure that it feels relaxed and squishy. Be aware that tension can easily arrive if you are not bringing enough weight onto the forearms. Do not lift legs up in this instance, as it may cause tension in the neck.

Shoulder Stand

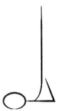

In shoulder stand, feel as the head goes on the floor that it is straight above the 'flagpole' and the neck is relaxed. As you come up into shoulder stand, check that there is no tension caused in the lifting up of the body. Use your core more if there is.

Once in shoulder stand, if tension in the neck, throat or palate is detected, begin to remember the isometric moves above, especially the one where you pushed the head into the ground and then released. Feel this area release and relax.

Plough

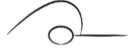   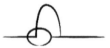

If the neck is relaxed, then you should find that the Plough feels easier to do; that there is less tension in the back of the legs and that it feels comfortable enough to hold for longer than is usual.

Standing Leg Raise

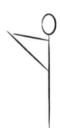

As you stand, gently take the weight over to one side of the body, ready to pick up one leg. As you begin to lift the leg, make sure that the core is engaged and that the lifting is not coming from your neck. Bring the knee up first and then extend the leg in front of you making sure that you are not tensing in the neck as you do so.

The Dancer

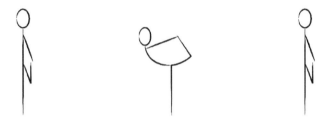

As you bring one leg behind you and you are stretching the thigh, check that you are not leaning forward just yet. Once the thigh has warmed up, pivot forward lifting the leg behind you as far as you feel is comfortable to do so. Check your head position – check where you are looking. Looking up or down can unbalance you, keep your eyes centred and your head in a neutral position, neither up nor down but relaxed.

TLR IN YOGA PRACTICE

Having integrated the TLR, now it is possible to use this new pattern in the neck for more effective yoga practice. As necks are tender and easily overstretched, it is important to emphasise that all yoga should be done with great awareness and self-control. There is no need to push to the edges of the stretches, just having an awareness of what is happening is often enough.

It is also a good idea to keep recalling the integration exercises regularly, as necks can easily tense up again once movement is introduced. More than any of the Reflexes, with the TLR we must maintain a relaxed pattern in the neck, or the neck may easily seize up. This can happen in class but most often it happens afterwards and if you are a teacher, you may not know about it. Therefore, it is often a good idea to remind yourself of this if you are going to do these exercises before any class. If you do get a crook neck by accident, do see it as a positive outcome. It means what you are doing is working and the Reflexes are releasing and doing the job they are meant to do.

I have found that if you work on the TLR too soon, all the work is quickly undone or doesn't last very long. So, necks take time and should be one of the Reflexes you tackle after a long period of work on the other Reflexes.

METHOD 1 – TAKING ADVANTAGE OF THE RELAXED FEELING IN THE NECK

Often yoga is practiced with emphasis on large muscle groups and stronger stretch sensations. With this method, we are trying to keep the neck in a relaxed position, and observing the subtle effect of this on the rest of the body your body. It is much harder to do, but by now, having had experience with the other Reflex work, you should be able to manage this with no problem.

For example, in Downward Dog

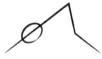

Come into a Downward Dog position and allow the head to be as loose as possible and gently look up and down, trying to keep the neck as relaxed as possible so that it is independent of the spine. Then recall an integration exercise like the flagpole and rag exercise. In this position, it is also very good to physically repeat this exercise in miniature movements. Once the integration exercise is complete, and as it integrates again in your body, observe not just what is happening in your neck but in the whole of the back body. Having a loose and relaxed neck can change how the shoulders move, how the lower back feels and even how effectively the hamstrings release.

Other examples that are good for this method are:

Triangle Forward Bend

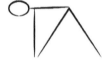

Behind the Back Prayer Forward Bend

METHOD 2 – COUNTERING PUSHING PATTERNS

As mentioned above, when working so deeply with the neck patterns, it is good to be cautious. This is why working on the floor is so good. Usually during a yoga class working with TLR, it does not take long before you can see on the faces of the students that they are struggling to stay upright and would rather be lying down. For this reason, lying down and practicing yoga is recommended for the TLR.

A good starting point is to remind yourself of the isometric integration exercises when doing floor work. Enquire as to whether when you practice certain asanas you find your head automatically pushing in certain directions and then remember the isometric integration exercise which is opposite to the pushing.

For example – Shoulder Stand

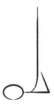

As you come into shoulder stand, before you are even up in the air, see if you can feel yourself pushing into the floor or into the air in front of you. Investigate what you do naturally so that there is some preparation for what comes next. It is very common for people to push hard into the floor beneath them when in shoulder stand. The neck can be tense, so remember to push into the 'invisible' hand on your forehead will help to correct this quickly and bring great relief.

Other poses where this works well are:

Plough

Fish

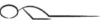

METHOD 3 – POSTURAL POSITIONING

Another good use for the TLR is to educate the body about how the head positioning affects the asanas. If you tend to push in certain directions (as above), it is important to keep reminding the body how it feels when the head finally finds a good position. So, you can ask yourself to explore a posture with the head too far forward, or too far back. You can do some integration exercises (head rolling is good) and then find the place where the head is neither too forward nor too back, 'just right' and work from there. Keep reminding yourself to find this good positioning and to keep the head where it feels just right, repeatedly. Habits are hard to break so you may find that you need to ask someone to give you a hand to align the head with your spine numerous times.

For example – Seated Half Twist

Come into the Seated Half Twist and try to gently move your head back and forth a few times, having a memory of one of the integration exercises (chose one you haven't used yet).

Then bring your head to where you feel is the central point, where the head feels most comfortable, where you feel it is straight above the spine. Look in a mirror and see if you are slightly off. If so, move your head very, very gently. Self-adjusting of head positions is a very good habit to get into when doing asanas.

Other poses that this works well in are:

Staff Pose

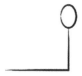

Forward Bends

Side Stretches

Balance Poses

CONCLUSION

This is the final piece in a very big jigsaw that we have covered in this book. There are many more minor Reflexes we have not covered which also affect our bodies and our neurology. As this Reflex is at the top of our 'tree' we have had to tackle it with sensitivity and caution and move slowly with it. The results of this work however will have an effect all the way down our 'tree' and now that we have the final piece of the jigsaw, it helps us to see the bigger picture of how well the body functions when all the different Reflexes are working well together.

If you have reached this far with the Reflex work, you will be reaping the benefits in areas you haven't even noticed yet. Those around you may remember how you used to be, but like a child, you have progressed through your neurological integration in a way that is almost invisible to you.

ONLY EXISTING

Sometimes I am suspended
between the dead
and the living.

A momentary speck of peace.

I have fled where
there are no demands
and I am free.

Only existing

I am suspended
between the ebb
and flow of existence.

A single stillness enveloping

I am no more,
no notions of self,
liberated.

Only existing

Sometimes I am free

of this body

of this mind.

A momentary release from desire.

I am suspended where

I no longer am

nor wish to be.

Free (of existing)

Veronika Peña de la Jara

CONCLUSION

I hope that all these ideas have sparked in you a joy of movement. I hope that you have seen what is possible with the integration of Primitive Reflexes, that you can relearn how to bring your body back to its best self.

The body will integrate itself first and slowly, without you realising probably, you will begin to see changes in your life you didn't think possible. Like watching a child grow day to day, you may not see the difference immediately, yet one day you will find yourself on the top of a rope walk in the jungle and remember that once, you could not have been there without fear or anxiety or vertigo.

Slowly, over time, as you work more and more and your plans come to fruition or your relationships improve, you will perhaps give credit to the work you have done here.

So many times, I have quietly congratulated my own clients as they pass their driving tests or GCSEs, lose weight or begin to thrive. It may be a few months or even a year or so later, yet I know a part of this change has come due to the work we did together. It can be thankless work, yet I am not in it for the praise. It is enough for me to know, quietly and late at night, that a difference has been made and that the message about the importance of the Primitive Reflex system in Integrating Trauma, continues to spread.

THE INVITATION

This mist, coats the ice trees ahead,
Showing me a narrow path
I have always known.

Today, I have used my newborn legs,
Climbed high upon the unexpected hill
And found a beautiful perspective instead.

The invitation, to step off the path ahead
Into a world of wonder and delight
Is the longing of the self for itself.

Little did I know, stuck beneath the clouds,
That on my misty path,
The sun shone anew each day.

The light, upon the mist below
Shines divine wonder
I have always known.

Today, I have my eyes peeled open,
Worked hard to break free of the trusted road ahead.
I have found a new perspective instead.

The invitation, to struggle for true purpose

Into a love, wildly in growth
is to step up towards curious faith.

Little did I know, working quietly away with meaning
That unexpectedly high above the hill
I'd see such an inspiring life ahead.

Veronika Peña de la Jara

BIBLIOGRAPHY

Beyond the Sea Squirt: A Journey with the Reflexes by Moira Dempsey

Integrating Reflexes through Play and Exercises: An interactive guide by Kokeb Girma McDonald

1. Moro Reflex
2. Spinal Galant
3. Asymmetrical Tonic Neck Reflex
4. Symmetrical Tonic Neck Reflex
5. Tonic Labyrinthine Reflex

The Rhythmic Movement Method: A Revolutionary Approach to Improved Health and Wellbeing by Harald Bloomberg.

Movements that Heal by Harald Bloomberg

Reflexes, Learning and Behavior: A Window into the Child's Mind: A Non-Invasive Approach to Solving Learning & Behavior Problems by Sally Goddard.

Attention, Balance and Coordination – The ABC of Learning, Sally Goddard, (2004).

The Well-Balanced Child, Sally Goddard (2004), UK Hawthorne Press.

A User's Guide to The Brain by Dr. John J. Ratey (2003).

Smart Moves: Why learning is not all in your head by Carla Hannaford (1995).

Awakening the Child's Heart by Carla Hannaford.

The Symphony of Reflexes: Interventions for Human Development, Autism, ADHD, CP, and Other Neurological Disorders by Bonnie Brandes.

Hackney, Peggy (2002) Making Connections, New York USA Routledge.

Hartley, Linda (1995) Wisdom of the Body Moving, Berkeley CA USA North Atlantic Books.

Koester, Cecilia (2006) Movement-Based Learning for Children of All Abilities, Reno, NV USA Movement Based Learning Inc.

Melillo, Robert and Leifman Gerry (2009): Neurobehavioral Disorders of Childhood: An Evolutionary Perspective, NY Springer.

Upledger, John (2010): A Brain is Born: Exploring the Birth and Development of the Central Nervous System, North Atlantic Books.

Dennison Paul & Gail: Eduk for Kids

Dennison Paul & Gail: Brain Gym, Teacher's Edition

Promislow, Sharon: Making the Brain, Body Connection.

O'Dell, Nancy & Cook, Patricia: Stopping Hyperactivity.

RESEARCH PAPERS ON REFLEXES AND NEUROLOGY

Mats Lindqvist & Greta Pettersson, "Rhythmical Movement Therapy with Chronic Schizophrenic patients," *Examensarbete 20 Poang*, Umea University 1993.

Svetlanda Masgutova with Nelly Akhmatova, "Integration of Dynamic and Postural Reflexes into the Whole-Body Movement System," Warsaw 2004.

Paul Dennison Ph D, "Total Core Repatterning and Movement Re-education," Edu-K Workshops, Ventura CA

McPhillips M, Heper P.G., Mulhem M: "Effects of Replicating Primary Reflex Movements on Specific Reading Difficulties in Children: A randomised, double blind, controlled trial," *The Lancet*, vol.355, No 9203, Pages 537-541.

McPhillips M & Jordan-Black J A: Primary Reflex Persistence in Children with Reading Difficulties (Dyslexia): A cross-sectional study," Neuropsychologia 2007, 45 pages 748-754.

Brewer, Chris and Campbell, Don G (1991). Rhythms of Learning, Tucson AS USA, Zephyr Press Inc.

Goldberg, Elkhonon: The Executive Brain – Frontal Lobes and the Civilised Mind. Oxford University Press, New York 2001

Martin JP: The Basal Ganglia and Posture, Pitman Medical Publishing, London 1967

Mary Gazca, Rebooting Development with A Rhythmic Motor Intervention, –- Unpublished Research Paper Dissertation, St Catherine's University, Minneapolis, MN USA (2012).

Tessa M. Grigg, The Voice of Parents Who Have Used Rhythmic Movement Training with Their Child– (2016).

Tessa Grigg, Wendy Fox-Turnbull and Ian Culpan, "Retained Primitive Reflexes: Perceptions of Parents Who Have Used Rhythmic Movement Training with Their Children," Journal of Child Healthcare, March 2018.

Listening, Auditory Processing, Reflex Links and Support with RMT, by Evonne Bennell (2016).

Dyslexia, RMT and Reflexes, by Moira Dempsey (2015).

Rhythmic Movement Training (RMTi) works with Rhythmic Movement Disorder (RMD) – Moira Dempsey (2015).

Rhythmic Movement Training (RMTi) and Working with Autism Spectrum Disorder (ASD) – Moira Dempsey.

Brown CG. Improving Fine Motor Skills in Young Children: An intervention study. *Educational Psychology in Practice* 2010; 26(3): 269-278.

McPhillips M, Jordan-Black J A. The Effect of Social Disadvantage on Motor Development in Young Children: A comparative study. *Journal of Child Psychology and Psychiatry* 2007; 48(12): 1214-1222.

Jordan-Black J A. The Effects of the Primary Movement Program on the Academic Performance of Children Attending Ordinary Primary School. *Journal of Research in Special Educational Needs* 2005; 5(3): 101-111.

McPhillips M, Sheehy N. Prevalence of Persistent Primary Reflexes and Motor Problems in Children with Reading Difficulties *Dyslexia* 2004; 10(4): 316-338.

McPhillips M. The Role of Persistent Primary Reflexes in Reading Delay. *Dyslexia Review* 2001; 13(1): 4-7.

McPhillips M, Hepper PG, Mulhern G. Effects of Replicating Primary Reflex Movements on Specific Reading Difficulties in Children. *Lancet* 2000; 355: 537-541.

Many, many more here:

https://rhythmicmovement.org/resources?fbclid=IwAR3E1yrSlB-gX8ooPwtvUL_DH2Xw1jSxS2Bjlf_eEAUFeOOTz_EfRX529FU

ABBREVIATIONS

AONB – Area of Outstanding Natural Beauty

ASD – Autism Spectrum Disorder

ATNR – Asymmetric Tonic Neck Reflex

BWY – British Wheel of Yoga

CNS – Central Nervous System

FHF – Foot Hand Face Reflex

FPR – Fear Paralysis Reflex

SGR – Spinal Galant Reflex

STNR – Symbiotic Tonic Neck Reflex

TLR – Tonic Labyrinthic Neck Reflex

RESOURCES

My website can be found at **https://the-empowered-feminine. co.uk**

My book and video courses can be found here to purchase. I also offer yoga classes online and one to one alongside body-based empowerment coaching sessions.

You can also subscribe to my blog on this site.

You can email me at **veronika@the-empowered-feminine. co.uk**

Facebook Page: Veronika Peña Jara

Instagram: the.empowered.feminine

Useful websites:
www.yotism.com/reflexyoga
www.rhythmicmovement.org
www.sallygoddardblythe.co.uk/school-programme

ACKNOWLEDGEMENTS

During a lifetime, every small step forward is facilitated by those around you. From your very first steps holding your parents' hands, to the mentors that help you leap forward as an adult, I am eternally grateful to you all. There are so many meditation teachers, yoga teachers, therapists and coaches that I am indebted to. I hope that you know that my work, as it reaches more and more people, would not have happened without you all.

My first thanks must go to my loving family, my daughter Isis and sons Eiran, Rafael and Kiyan, who have steadfastly stood by my side, helping me by either being my guinea pigs or by reading these words or editing videos, with many cups of tea to boot. Your relentless cheering me on has helped me keep my eye on the ball. All of this was brought forward to aid your generation, so that you did not have to stay in any trauma for long.

My mother, who has always expressed nothing but pride in anything I do, even the less understandable decisions I have made. Thank you for your unwavering support and love.

My father, who's loving hand and questioning look, always kept me centred and gave me great holidays, where I could recover from life. I am so grateful.

Again, I must thank Nicole Zimbler, my sister in learning, without whom the idea and development of Reflex Yoga may never have come about. It is due to her curiosity and intuitiveness that I embarked on this journey of uniting Primitive Reflexes and Yoga. I am forever grateful for the direction my life took with you in it.

I have many friends. However, a few have been there for me at my lowest, darkest moments and have always had faith I would pull through and thrive. Thank you, Raquel Faraco, Joy Minton, Holly Winner and Rosie Evans. My life is full of fun, food and frolics because of you girls!

I have had a string of dedicated meditation teachers of the Dhamma.org tradition, I am grateful to each one of the line of teachers that brought the jewel of Dhamma to me.

To all the yogis who have inspired my practice, from my first now forgotten Iyengar teacher in Reading, through to Jay Rossi of Kashmir Yoga and then to Nicole of Yotism and beyond. I thank all my yogi friends who I have practiced, collaborated with and laughed with at many yoga festivals over the years. Every one of you has given me a new jewel to add to my treasure chest. Thank you all.

I thank all my long-suffering yoga students, who have patiently helped me develop this technique, especially in the early years when it was not well formed. They say a yoga teacher improves with teaching, I reinvented myself a few times, so I did start from the beginning a few times too. Some of my classes may well have been disjointed and too wordy as I tried to integrate what I knew in my head into my body. Thank you for your patience and for your inspiration. Every time I see the look of acknowledgement, of understanding, of awareness in the body, I am humbled.

ABOUT THE AUTHOR

Veronika has been a yoga teacher for 25 years. She is a yoga teacher trainer and specialises in many areas of yoga: early years, pregnancy, mother and child, children, teen and adult yoga. She is a yoga teacher trainer in the Reflex Yoga method with Nicole Zimbler at Yotism.

Veronika came across yoga when she was working in Thailand as a dive master.

She trained to be a yoga teacher with the British School of Yoga in 1999 and went on to do further training in other related areas like Thai Chi and meditation.

She has been a keen Vipassana meditator since 1999. She practices this technique every day and attends 10-day silent retreats at least once a year.

Reflex Yoga is the brainchild of Veronika's and Nicole Zimbler's lifetime work. It is born of Veronika's natural ability to develop a Yoga method alongside Nicole's massive knowledge of the Reflex System, which Veronika has also studied extensively.

Veronika undertook further training in two modalities that she now incorporates into her work. The first is Melanie Tonia Evans's work in NARP and the second is Claire Zammit's work of Evolving Wisdom.

Melanie's work taught Veronika about Empowerment from within – how to create personal boundaries and resource herself. This was the final push out of trauma after years of preparation with Reflex Yoga.

Claire Zammit's work was the final piece of the jigsaw that made sense of everything she had learnt thus far. when she first heard Claire speak about what Feminine Power is, she was inspired to use it in her own life and bring it into her teaching.

Claire's ability to bring her message across so clearly has recently inspired Veronika to become a speaker to bring her knowledge to the world. She is currently embarking on a Stage Speaker Training with Sage Lavine of Women Rocking Business.

Milton Keynes UK
Ingram Content Group UK Ltd.
UKHW030746081024
449420UK00011B/238